For Elsevier:

Commissioning Editor: Rita Demetriou-Swanwick
Development Editor: Catherine Jackson
Project Manager: Kerrie-Anne Jarvis
Design Direction: George Ajayi
Illustrations Manager: Merlyn Harvey
Illustrator: Graeme Chambers

Wellbeing in Dementia

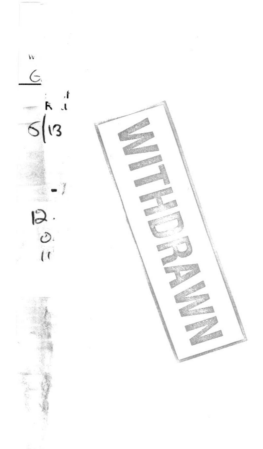

Wellbeing in Dementia

An occupational approach for therapists and carers

Second Edition

Tessa Perrin PhD, MSc, DipCOT
Independent Occupational Therapist and Director, Occupation Matters

Hazel May MA, DipCOT, SROT
Practice Development Consultant and Trainer, University of Bradford, Bradford Dementia Group

Elizabeth Anderson BA (Hons), MSc, DPhil
University Teacher, University of Bradford, Bradford Dementia Group

Foreword by

Dawn Brooker PhD, CPsychol, (clin) AFBPsS
Professor of Dementia Care Practice and Research, University of Bradford, Bradford Dementia Group

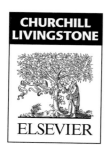

CHURCHILL
LIVINGSTONE

ELSEVIER

EDINBURGH LONDON NEW YORK OXFORD PHILADELPHIA ST LOUIS SYDNEY TORONTO 2008

CHURCHILL
LIVINGSTONE
ELSEVIER

First edition 2000
Second edition 2008
  Reprinted 2009

ISBN: 978 0 443 10399 5

British Library Cataloguing in Publication Data
A catalogue record for this book is available from the British Library.

Library of Congress Cataloging in Publication Data
A catalog record for this book is available from the Library of Congress.

Notice
Neither the Publisher nor the Authors assume any responsibility for any loss or injury and/or damage to persons or property arising out of or related to any use of the material contained in this book. It is the responsibility of the treating practitioner, relying on independent expertise and knowledge of the patient, to determine the best treatment and method of application for the patient.

The Publisher

Printed in China

Contents

Foreword

Wellbeing in Dementia

This is an important book. It was important when it came out in its first edition and its central message is still as fresh in this second edition. It is written by three women who in their own quiet way have played an enormous part in the way we conceptualise modern dementia care.

In these pages you will find a wealth of ways to challenge outdated assumptions about dementia and a therapeutic approach to promote wellbeing. Therapeutic nihilism towards dementia has no place here. The work is scholarly and provides a theoretical and conceptual underpinning for why wellbeing in dementia is promoted as a key outcome. From a practice point of view it is grounded in many case studies that those working directly with people with dementia will instantly recognise.

The additional material in this edition helps to clarify our understanding of the personal experience of dementia. People with dementia often suffer most when their behaviour and responses to their situation are misunderstood and misattributed. This book provides a number of interlinking models and frameworks to assist understanding.

Although this book has particular relevance for occupational therapists, there is so much within its pages that will appeal to a much wider audience. Commissioners of services, managers, educators, trainers as well as professionally qualified practitioners from all disciplines will find much here that will help them support the work of those delivering direct care. It is a practical book, written with great humanity that has the ability to change hearts and minds.

This book frees its readers to be creative and playful in the way in which we think about occupation and well-being. These chapters should be compulsory reading for all those involved in the organisation of activities for people with dementia. The chapters on the significance of the carer and non-verbal communication should be compulsory reading for all those involved in care and support. As part of the working group for the English National Dementia Strategy I have been involved in many discussions about the core competencies for those who work directly with people with dementia. The final chapter in this book on the role of the dementia therapist sets out these competencies beautifully.

When the first edition of this book appeared I believe it was way ahead of its time. I welcome this new edition as being of its time. It will be read by those thirsty for ways of working with people with dementia to help them live their lives despite of a diagnostic label that many people still see as signifying the end of a life worth living. This book is about life. Grab it with both hands.

Dawn Brooker PhD, CPsychol, (clin) AFBPsS
Professor of Dementia Care Practice and Research
University of Bradford
Bradford Dementia Group

Preface to 2nd edition

It is now some seven years since the first edition of this book went on the bookshelves. As we came to prepare the manuscript for the second edition we were reminded of our closing words to the original, in which we hoped that in ten years time advances in the fields of dementia care and occupational therapy would have made the book redundant. There have, of course, been considerable advances in both fields generally during that time, but none which we feel renders this book redundant, and so we decided to proceed.

Canvassing opinion from our colleagues on the need for this text to remain in print, one colleague who is very active in education and research made a helpful comment. She said that when guiding students and others towards essential reading in the occupation and dementia field, there was a range of texts she would recommend. But for those wanting a sound theoretical underpinning to the field, she would always highlight *Wellbeing in Dementia*. This has been a helpful insight which confirms our own feelings about the book. It was always intended to be a contribution to theory, a frame of reference which would serve to guide practice. It is pleasing that some still perceive it in this way. Over the years we have had a fair bit of feedback; none of it has been negative and nobody has challenged our propositions. We had expected some disagreement and had in some measure looked forward to some healthy debate, but it hasn't come our way. So maybe we need to assume that the greater number of our readers is in accord with our ideas. This too has encouraged us to feel that the book should remain available.

The essence of the book remains the same, but there are two key changes. Chapters 1 and 9 have been overhauled and updated. Thinking on the nature of dementia itself moves on apace and we were aware that we needed an abler brain to bring us up to speed. We are delighted therefore to welcome Dr Elizabeth Anderson's contribution in Chapter 1. This has given us a succinct, up-to-date statement on dementia which addresses with clarity the neurological/psychological debate. Chapter 9, reflecting the developments in assessment practice which have taken place over the intervening years, has also been revised. From her extensive experience in research and practice development, Hazel May has reviewed the assessment tools now available and has offered a model for assessment which reflects current thinking on the measurement of wellbeing and engagement in dementia care.

And so we edge towards an ever greater clarity and excellence in our dealings with the procedures and practices of dementia care. We have worked in the dementia care field now for well over 20 years, and have to say that it has been a great privilege to be a part of the wave of seminal development which has been gathering momentum over that time. Since the first edition was published, both Hazel and Tessa have been overtaken by a personal experience of dementia in the context of our respective families –altogether different of course, from dealing with dementia as a professional. It has been an experience which has taken us both to the edge, but a salutary experience nevertheless. We have both found ourselves grateful for the knowledge, the experience and the contacts we have acquired over our years in dementia care. This has made the undertaking of the carer role a little easier, but even with this as a foundation we have found that the experience has stretched us almost to our limits, and we have wondered what on earth it must be like for those coming to the experience without the 'preparation' that we have had. This further challenges our continued commitment to this field of work, to support, educate and provide for those living with dementia who have not had the privilege of the insights we have gained. The need remains urgent, the task remains vast: we commend our new edition to the continued endeavour.

Tessa Perrin
Hazel May
Elizabeth Anderson
2008

Chapter 1

Understanding dementia

INTRODUCTION

The question 'What is dementia?' is easy to ask and hard to answer. It may be easier to begin with what dementia is not. One thing that dementia is not, and has never been defined to be, is a disease. Rather, dementia has always been defined to be a syndrome of intellectual decline. 'Syndrome' sounds daunting but all it means is 'a collection of symptoms'. These symptoms are usually some or all of the following:

- memory loss
- language difficulties
- difficulties with spatial awareness and skilled movement
- a loss of knowledge and understanding of the world
- problems with reasoning, planning and judgement
- changes in personality, behaviour and emotional control.

Even these sub-categories are quite broad and cover a lot of different specific problems and difficulties and there is considerable variation from one person to the next in the particular mix of symptoms they experience. The aim of this chapter is to explain what dementia is and what causes it. To work successfully with people with dementia it is important to have a sound understanding of the condition they are living with. As part of this explanation, the chapter will outline the basic organisation of the human brain and reveal the parts that are most vulnerable and least vulnerable to damage in dementia. This provides a basis not only for understanding why certain symptoms are common amongst people with dementia, but also for why we need to recognise the individuality of the person with dementia. It is important that we do not assume that the dementia is simply 'global intellectual decline' but undertake a careful assessments of both lost and preserved abilities in a person with dementia. The chapter will also explain why brain damage must be set in a wider context that covers the person's past and present circumstances. The chapter will show how we can use knowledge about the brain, and in particular the organisation of memory functions, to move into the mind of the person with dementia and take on their perspective of the world. This perspective is central to understanding the needs and behaviour of a person with dementia and providing care that promotes their wellbeing.

WHAT IS DEMENTIA?

The current definition of dementia by the World Health Organization (1993), in the 10th edition of its International Classification of Diseases (ICD-10), is:

> *'A syndrome due to disease of the brain, usually of a chronic or progressive nature, in which there is disturbance of multiple higher cortical functions, including memory, thinking, orientation, comprehension, calculation, learning capacity, language and judgement. Consciousness is not clouded. The impairments of cognitive function are commonly accompanied, and occasionally preceded, by deterioration in emotional control, social behaviour or motivation. This syndrome occurs in Alzheimer's disease, in cerebrovascular disease, and in other conditions primarily or secondarily affecting the brain.'*

This definition makes it clear that the core symptoms of dementia (that is, the problems with memory, the confusion, the difficulties with language and understanding, the changes in emotion and behaviour) are primarily due to damage to the brain. The above definition also makes clear that there are many different challenges to the brain that can cause the symptoms of dementia. Thus, the word 'dementia' does not refer to a specific disease, but rather is an umbrella term which covers many different forms of disease and damage to the brain that affect its 'higher' or 'cognitive' functions. The most common causes of dementia are summarised in Table 1.1.

Table 1.1   A summary of the most common causes of dementia

Common primary causes	Common secondary causes
Alzheimer's disease	Vitamin B deficiency
Vascular dementia	Hypothyroidism
Lewy body dementia	Depression
Frontotemporal dementia	

Some of these causes affect the brain directly (primary causes) whilst others are indirect (secondary causes). Secondary causes cause some kind of disruption to normal processing within the brain but do not damage the structure of the brain. Because the structure of the brain has not been damaged these dementias can often be reversed through successful treatment of the underlying condition. Table 1.1 shows that the most common secondary causes are vitamin B deficiency, hypothyroidism and depression. For people with secondary dementia the prognosis is good and they do not face the long-term challenges associated with the primary dementias.

The focus of this book is to improve the prospects for quality of life and wellbeing for those with primary dementia, for whom the prognosis is more challenging. These are the dementias that directly damage the brain and are irreversible and usually progressive. The most common form of primary dementia is Alzheimer's disease (accounting for 50–60% of all dementias). Alzheimer's disease is a neurodegenerative disease that slowly strips cells out of the most developed parts of the brain. The usual duration of the disease is 4–6 years, although there is huge variation, with some people dying within a year or two and others experiencing a gentler trajectory of decline that can span over two decades (Corey-Bloom & Fleisher 2005). The disease is recognised at post-mortem by its hallmarks, senile plaques and neurofibrillary tangles, within the brain tissue. In recent years much has been learnt about this disease, but it is a complex process and debate continues about what causes it: whether the plaques and tangles cause cell death, or whether they are simply the only visible by-products of dysfunctional cellular processes that have yet to be revealed and understood (for a review see Whalley 2001).

Cerebrovascular damage (vascular dementia) is also a significant cause of dementia, accounting for about 20% of all dementias. The term vascular dementia covers all dementias which are primarily caused by a problem with the blood supply to the brain. The most common form is multi-infarct dementia, a condition in which the person develops a vulnerability to tiny strokes (sometimes called 'mini strokes' or 'strokelets'). In the early stages the brain damage that results from these small strokes is too minimal to cause any noticeable change to the person's skills and intellect, but as the damage accumulates the symptoms of dementia emerge and develop.

Other recently recognised significant causes of dementia are Lewy body dementia and frontotemporal dementia. Like Alzheimer's disease, these are both neurodegenerative processes that progressively kill brain cells. The causes and mechanisms of these processes, like those of Alzheimer's disease, remain only partially understood. The process underlying Lewy body dementia leaves a different pathological hallmark within affected nerve cells – the Lewy body, a small, spherical deposit of insoluble protein. Post-mortem studies have revealed that Lewy body disease and Alzheimer's disease often exist together. Indeed, mixed causes of dementia, sometimes called 'the mixed dementias', are common (Esiri et al 2001). The processes underlying the frontotemporal dementias are recognised by the very severe atrophy, or thinning, of brain tissue in the frontal and temporal lobes of the brain (key areas of the brain which will be introduced and explained in the latter half of this chapter). Pick's disease is a particular form of frontotemporal dementia, again recognised at post-mortem by a particular neuropathological hallmark within damaged cells called the Pick body.

If you wish to learn more about the nature of these diseases, the best place to start is the Alzheimer's Society website which has an excellent factsheet about each one. Were you to delve into medical textbooks on the topic you would find that whilst these are the major causes of dementia there are numerous other rare causes of primary dementia, including Creutzfelt–Jakob disease. It is possible to generate lists of causes with over 50 entries but taken together the rare causes account for only 1–2% of all primary dementias.

It remains impossible to diagnose the underlying cause of a primary dementia with 100% accuracy. There are no clinical tests that can confirm that the pathology of Alzheimer's disease, Lewy body disease or frontotemporal dementia is developing within a person's brain. Vascular dementia is related to general indices of vascular health (e.g. diabetes, high cholesterol and high blood pressure) but these are remote indices and do not give a precise indication of the degree to which the brain may be affected by vascular damage. Each form of dementia has characteristics which help clinicians to make a diagnosis of cause (see Table 1.2 below), but there is much variation and overlap in how all these conditions manifest, meaning that in some cases it is impossible to be sure what is causing the dementia.

With the neurodegenerative conditions (Alzheimer's disease, Lewy body disease and frontotemporal dementia) the progression of symptoms is usually continual, but Lewy body dementia and frontotemporal dementia tend to progress at a faster rate than Alzheimer's disease. Lewy body disease is associated with more day to day fluctuations, more of a 'good-day, bad-day' pattern, than Alzheimer's disease, whilst vascular dementia often has a 'stop-start' or 'stepwise' pattern to the progression, each step down representing the occurrence of a new 'mini-stroke'. These characteristics have been incorporated into diagnostic guidelines which are recognised internationally (Table 1.2). Such developments represent significant progress from the days when a general diagnosis of dementia was considered sufficient and was often applied without diagnostic rigour to explain any situation in which an elderly person's behaviour appeared to depart from the norm. Nonetheless, there is still much work to be done in finding the markers that will allow clinicians to make an early and accurate diagnosis of cause.

With respect to the specific symptoms of the different primary dementias, it is worth noting that the symptom profile for dementia as a general syndrome has been strongly influenced by the specific symptoms of Alzheimer's disease. Because Alzheimer's disease is the most common cause of dementia, the stereotype of dementia is driven by the characteristics of this particular disease. This has over-shadowed the fact that the less common causes have slightly different symptom profiles. Thus, whilst memory loss is a central feature of Alzheimer's disease, because this particular disease process is focused in the parts of the brain essential for memory function, it is a less prominent feature of the other forms of dementia, where the damage may be focused in other areas of the brain. Vascular damage can strike anywhere within the brain, meaning that the pattern

Table 1.2 Summary of the key characteristics of the four main causes of primary dementia

Cause (Key Diagnostic Guideline)	Characteristics
Alzheimer's disease McKhann et al (1984)	Memory loss is first symptom and dominates symptom profile during early years Loss of abilities is gradual but continual
Vascular dementia Roman et al (1993) Chui et al (1992)	Memory loss is probable but does not dominate the symptom profile Loss of abilities more 'patchy' depending upon where exactly mini-strokes occur May be early loss of more basic sensory and motor functions Exists alongside signs of poor vascular health (high blood pressure, high cholesterol etc.)
Lewy body dementia McKeith et al (1996)	Fluctuating cognitive ability Visual hallucinations Parkinsonian symptoms
Frontotemporal dementia The Lund and Manchester Group (1994)	Changes in either (a) personality, social and emotional control or (b) language are more dominant than, and precede, memory loss

of symptoms that occurs in vascular dementia may be more random and include more basic problems with sensory and motor functions (e.g. visual field cuts, poor gait, muscle weakness, stuttering speech, general motor slowing/clumsiness, incontinence) even when the intellectual problems, which are the core of the dementia syndrome, remain relatively mild.

Frontotemporal dementia is focused (as its name suggests) in the frontal lobe and temporal lobe of the brain, regions that are essential for social and emotional control. Memory is usually retained in the early stages of this disorder, but there are drastic changes to personality and behaviour, with behaviour becoming impulsive, reckless and inconsiderate. Often this condition is confused with functional psychiatric conditions and is not recognised as being a form of organic brain disease. This creates particular difficulties for the person and their family because it is assumed that the change in personality and behaviour is a functional problem (that is, something wrong with the person's mind or attitude) when in reality the cause is an aggressive form of brain damage that is quite beyond the person's control.

Turning finally to Lewy body disease, there is some overlap between this condition and Parkinson's disease. The symptom profile of Lewy body dementia often includes Parkinsonian features such as mask-like facial expressions, a shuffling gait or tremors. This form of dementia is also associated with visual hallucinations and greater instability of cognitive function, periods of lucidity alternating with periods of deep confusion, as referred to above.

A careful medical history of the nature and onset of the symptoms of a dementia, combined with other essential investigations, such as blood tests to check for secondary causes and brain scans to check for strokes or tumours, usually leads to a correct diagnosis of the underlying cause. Post-mortem studies show that careful application of the diagnostic guidelines referenced above leads to high, but not perfect, accuracy rates (for review see Ballard & Bannister 2005). There is debate about whether dementia should be diagnosed (Drickamer & Lachs 1992). GPs face real anxieties in relation to diagnosing dementia (Downs 1996, Downs et al 2002) and many are reluctant to make a diagnosis, particularly directly to the person with dementia, on the grounds that a diagnosis is not helpful when there is so little that can be done to cure or treat the condition (Vassilas & Donaldson 1998, Renshaw et al 2001). However, there is evidence to suggest that a thorough investigation and diagnosis is helpful to people with dementia and their families, and there is growing agreement that the decision as to whether or not the diagnosis is given should lie with the person with dementia rather than the clinician (Meyers 1997). Being told that you have an irreversible and progressive brain disease is always going to be bad news, but identification of the cause can reassure people that there is a reason for the change and reduces stress (Audit Commission 2002).

Recent guidelines highlight the importance of early and accurate diagnosis in enabling people with dementia and their families to adapt (Department of Health 2001, National Institute for Clinical Excellence 2006, National Audit Office 2007). Furthermore, in the long-term, the development of cures or effective pharmacological treatments depends critically upon understanding and addressing the specific causes of dementia, and so it is vital that research into how to understand and detect the different forms of dementia continues. However, sadly, it is likely that cures for any of the common forms of dementia remain a long way off. In the meantime, for the person with dementia and those who care for that person, understanding **how to respond** to changes in memory, cognition and behaviour is of more central concern than understanding what is causing those changes. Regardless of underlying cause, the symptoms of dementia are best regarded as **cognitive disabilities**, challenges that require **adaptation and support**, rather than signs of a terminal and irreversible disease about which nothing can be done. The importance of adopting a positive attitude towards people with dementia will be discussed in more detail in the next section.

LIVING WITH PRIMARY DEMENTIA

Living with a primary dementia is extremely challenging. Because there is direct damage to the structure of the brain in primary dementia, these forms of dementia cannot be reversed, and pharmacological treatments are limited to the anti-dementia drugs. These drugs do not repair the damage to the structure of the brain, but seek to help the brain cells that remain to communicate effectively with one another by boosting levels of a key neurotransmitter called acetylcholine. These drugs have been shown to delay cognitive decline in Alzheimer's disease, but whilst the effect is reliable, the size of the effect is modest (Takeda et al 2006). The minimal size of the benefit has led to the recent decision of NICE to restrict prescription of these drugs on the NHS to those whose dementia is moderate (NICE, 2006). Those with mild dementia and severe dementia are not thought to benefit enough for the costs to be justified. The decision, however, is very controversial. Experts have questioned the clinical basis for the decision (it is very hard to give someone with mild Alzheimer's disease a diagnosis but tell them they must wait until they deteriorate further before they can be treated) and also the suitability of the cost–benefit analysis undertaken by NICE (O'Brien 2006). NICE's guidance has caused extreme anger amongst people with dementia and their families, and key charities, such as the Alzheimer's Society, have organised campaigns to get the decision reversed. The drug companies that produce the drugs have also challenged the guidance, leading to the first ever Judicial Review of a NICE decision. The Judicial Review concluded in August 2007 with a decision that changes to the guidelines were required regarding the use of the MMSE score (Folstein et al 1975) to ensure that the disability and race discrimination law is not breached, but that in other respects the NICE guidance was to be upheld, meaning that people with mild Alzheimer's disease will not have access to these drugs on the NHS. Neil Hunt, Chief Executive of the Alzheimer's Society, said in a statement on 27 September 2007 that the Society would not appeal against the decision, but reiterated that the guidance made no sense from a clinical, monetary or moral perspective.

As noted earlier, the lack of effective biomedical treatments for the causes of dementia has led many doctors and other health professionals to take a negative and pessimistic view of the condition (Audit Commission 2002, National Audit Office 2007). The belief that nothing can be done to help people with dementia contributes to the poor level of provision of services to help people with dementia live with the disabilities their brain damage causes, so it is vital that this belief is challenged. Furthermore, because the symptoms of dementia are within the realm of the intellect it is easy to overlook the fact that there is a physical cause for the symptoms. Damage to the parts of the brain that support memory will cause memory loss as surely as damage to the spinal cord will cause paralysis. Dementia does not operate within a 'mind realm' which is quite independent of the body and therefore subject to the law of 'mind over matter' rather than 'cause and effect'. Lecturing, disciplining, arguing with, pleading with, despairing of or drilling people with dementia with respect to forgotten facts and lost skills is not going to bring those skills back. **But this is not cause for pessimism**. There is a direct parallel with physical disabilities – **the extent to which a person is disabled by intellectual or cognitive disabilities depends to a large extent upon the level and quality of support that is provided to help them live with those disabilities.**

The answer to the negative view for the prospects for people with dementia is not to deny that they have a progressive and incurable condition, but rather to recognise that *progressive and incurable* is not synonymous with *hopeless and pointless*. It is possible to accept the reality of primary dementia and still be positive. Although it is not possible to cure dementia, it is possible to radically transform the nature of the care and support that is provided to those who are affected (Kitwood 1997, Brooker 2007). The more people see that people with dementia, when given the correct support and care, can live rewarding and happy lives, the less cause there will be for fear of the condition.

The remainder of this chapter will explain the nature of the neurological impairments of dementia in more detail in order to demonstrate that **personhood** (Rogers 1961, Kitwood 1997) that is, a person's subjective experience of having a sense of being, agency and unity as a unique human being, persists even when abilities such as memory, knowledge and language are lost. Loss of these so-called 'higher cognitive abilities' raises serious challenges to life, in particular dependency, but these losses do not rob a person of subjective existence. Memory and cognition are very important to our sense of self, and our expression of self, but the brain supports many other functions beyond memory and cognition and we are more than memory and cognition. Occupation and activities tailored to the person's remaining strengths are essential to a person's sense of wellbeing. Correct assessment of a person's abilities and disabilities requires both a general understanding of the organisation of functions within the brain, and an ability to apply that general knowledge to a particular individual through careful observation. This chapter will outline the general knowledge of the brain and its functions, which is required as an underpinning, whilst the remainder of the book will deal with the more complex task of assessing individuals and developing tailor-made strategies for individual people with dementia.

THE NATURE OF THE NEUROLOGICAL IMPAIRMENT

The vast majority of people you work with will have dementia because of underlying brain damage. This does not, however, mean that brain damage is the only thing influencing their experience and behaviour. A key purpose of this chapter is to explain how brain damage interacts with psychological factors (such as personality and life history) and social factors (attitudes to dementia, the behaviour of other people towards the person with dementia) in determining the expression of a person's dementia and their lived experience of that dementia.

Kitwood (1989, 1997) recognised a complex interplay between brain states and psychological states and stressed the importance of seeing neurological impairment (i.e. brain damage) as just one component of dementia. His position is elegantly captured in his equation:

D = NI + H + SP + B + P

(where D is dementia, NI is neurological impairment, H is health, SP is social psychology, B is biography and P is personality) and his aphorism that we must see:

the PERSON with dementia

not

the person with DEMENTIA.

Kitwood did not deny that neurological impairment is a key component of dementia, but was concerned that once a person received a diagnosis of dementia the attention of others became inappropriately focused upon the dementia and the problems it caused, such that the person fell out of the picture. The fact that the neurological impairment was occurring to a particular individual with a unique set of factors relating to their personality and experiences that could influence the expression and experience of their dementia was overlooked.

This raises some problems with explaining the nature of the neurological impairment that underpins dementia. With dementia being an umbrella concept having many possible underlying causes, it is impossible to be definitive about the nature of the neurological impairment. Each cause, as explained above, affects the brain differently. On top of that, each person with dementia is an individual and there will be differences even within a cause as to how that person's brain has been affected and damaged. Psychosocial factors, such as personality and life-history, add further variability in terms of how neurological impairment expresses itself. Kitwood's message that each person with dementia must be treated as an individual, and not as a generic instance of dementia, cannot be stressed strongly enough (Kitwood 1997). Nonetheless, there are broad principles that can be drawn out which are helpful for understanding the challenges people with dementia face as a consequence of their condition.

First, the core symptoms of dementia are associated with damage to a particular part of the brain called the cerebral cortex. The human brain is not a single structure but a whole nest of interacting structures. Different parts of the brain have evolved at different times and each structure has a specialised function within the brain's overall goal of regulating the body and behaviour to meet the needs and desires of its owner. The brain is divided into three main sections (hindbrain, midbrain and forebrain) with each section containing a cluster of individual structures. The structures of the hindbrain are found in the brain stem (Fig 1.1) which is an

Figure 1.1   A picture of the human brain showing how the cerebral cortex covers the whole outer surface of the two cerebral hemispheres of the forebrain and that there are many other subcortical structures lying below.

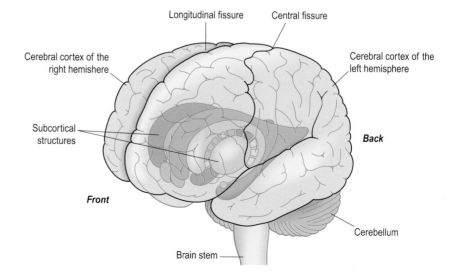

extension of the spinal cord. Structures of the midbrain, and in particular the forebrain, have become greatly enlarged during human evolution. Figure 1.1 also shows the cerebellum (part of the midbrain), a largish structure that sits at the back of the brain underneath the two enormous cerebral hemispheres that form the forebrain, the two hemispheres being divided by a deep cleft in the brain called the longitudinal fissure (also shown in Fig 1.1). The forebrain contains a multitude of structures, and of these the cerebral cortex is the largest.

Figure 1.1 shows that the cerebral cortex is a sheet of nerve cells that covers the entire outer surface of the two cerebral hemispheres that comprise the forebrain. The cortex is thin, but in terms of surface area, it is vast. If it were pulled off the surface and laid flat it would measure nearly a metre square. Within the sheet are millions upon millions of nerve cells, capable of making trillions upon trillions of connections with one another. These connections support the most advanced aspects of human intelligence, such as conscious perception, knowledge, reasoning and decision-making. However, the cortex can only achieve these amazing functions by working with the whole hierarchy of structures underlying it, going right back down to the humble body. Without the body the cortex would not know anything or be able to do anything. Without 'delegating' the more mechanical or procedural aspects of control to other structures in the brain and spinal cord it would be overwhelmed.

Figure 1.1 also shows that there are many subcortical structures lying beneath the cortex (in fact those illustrated are only a small portion of all those structures). In isolation from the subcortical structures that lie beneath it, the cerebral cortex, despite being phenomenally complex and powerful, could never do anything. It could be likened to a genius who sits in a study in his ivory tower generating excellent plans about how to order and improve his society. To achieve these plans he must listen to messengers coming from the outside world and employ workers to put his ideas into action. If he does not do these things, his ideas remain locked up in the tower and of no value to himself or anyone else.

The cerebral cortex, as noted above, is particularly vulnerable to damage by the causes of dementia, but many of the subcortical structures that lie beneath are not so badly affected, particularly during the mild to moderate phases of a dementia (although it is likely that there will be some degree of subcortical damage and that this will get worse as the condition progresses). With respect to the analogy above, the messengers are still bringing information in, and there are workers ready and able to do the work, but the plans they are working to are increasingly awry with respect to a full understanding of the world in which they are operating. It is with respect to this dynamic interplay between the most damaged and less damaged parts of the brain that the importance of attending to the psychosocial components of Kitwood's equation becomes apparent. The remainder of this section will detail the particular functions of different regions of the cortex to provide the foundation upon which such interactions between brain damage and psychological and social factors can be understood.

Damage to the cerebral cortex is not a simple phenomenon. The cortex has the overall job of supporting the 'higher' cognitive abilities, but these functions cover a huge range of specific abilities ranging from memory, through language, knowledge and spatial ability, to personality and social control. To support such a diverse range of functions the cortex itself is divided, with specific regions being responsible for specific abilities. Figure 1.2 shows that each half of the cerebral cortex (right and left) is divided into four lobes; the occipital, the temporal, the parietal and the frontal. The frontal lobe, as its name suggests, comprises the cortex covering the front of each cerebral hemisphere and is bounded by two more deep clefts in the brain, the central fissure which divides front from back and the Sylvian fissure which divides the two 'arms' of the brain which come down behind the ears.

The three other lobes (parietal, temporal and occipital) are found behind the central fissure (Fig 1.2). The occipital lobe is found at the very back of each cerebral hemisphere, whilst the parietal lobe is at the top of the brain, immediately behind the central fissure. The temporal lobe covers the 'arm' of brain that comes down behind the ear. You will see from Figure 1.2 that there is no clear boundary between the temporal, parietal and occipital lobes; they all merge into one another in the area at the top of the Sylvian fissure.

The division of the cortex into the four lobes is important because each lobe is involved in different aspects of the 'higher' cognitive abilities, as summarised in Table 1.3 and Figure 1.3. The broad function of each lobe will be discussed first, before presenting a more detailed account of the specific symptoms of dementia that are associated with damage to each lobe.

The occipital lobe is the smallest of the four lobes and, as noted above, is located at the very back of the cerebral hemispheres. The optic nerve sends information from the eye to this lobe and the whole lobe is dedicated to the processing of visual information. The networks of this lobe process light information to extract key features (edges, colours, movements etc.) and then use this information to build up a complex representation of the external world. This complex representation reveals what objects are

Figure 1.2 A picture of the human brain showing the four lobes of the left cerebral hemisphere and two of the right (the temporal and occipital are hidden from view).

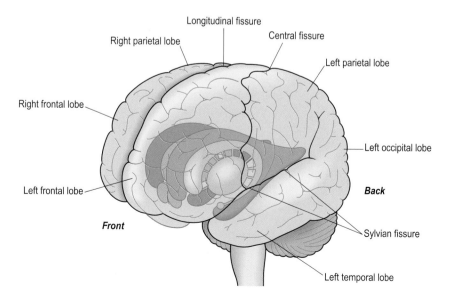

Table 1.3. Summary of the key functions of the four lobes of the cerebral cortex

Lobe	Function
Occipital lobe	Vision
Temporal lobe	Memory, language and understanding
Parietal lobe	Body control and space
Frontal lobe	Control of behaviour, planning, and decision-making

Figure 1.3 A picture showing the location and broad functions of the four lobes of the cerebral cortex.

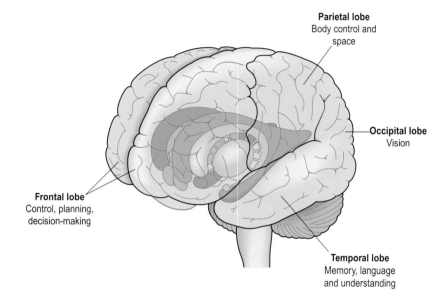

Parietal lobe
Body control and space

Occipital lobe
Vision

Frontal lobe
Control, planning, decision-making

Temporal lobe
Memory, language and understanding

present in the environment and what they are doing. The location of the occipital lobe right at the back of the brain places it in a protected position, and of all the lobes it is also the least vulnerable to damage. It is, therefore, unusual for the occipital lobe to be damaged in dementia [although in some forms of vascular dementia strokes may affect the region and cause a loss of vision on one side of space (hemianopia) or blind spots within the visual field]. In general this means that the basic ability to see the external world is usually not undermined in dementia.

However, whilst the occipital lobe tends not to be a focus of attack, the networks of the occipital lobe have limited power in terms of **interpreting** what is seen. Interpreting functions are served by networks in the **temporal** and **parietal lobes** which develop knowledge networks that allow people to understand what they see and to interact skillfully with the external environment. The occipital lobe sends the results of its visual analyses forward into the **temporal lobe** in order for **information** about what is seen to be accessed. The temporal lobe is very vulnerable to the causes of dementia (particularly Alzheimer's disease and frontotemporal dementia). Thus, whilst people with dementia continue to see normally, it becomes increasingly hard for them to **understand** what it is that they are seeing. The vast networks of nerve cells in the temporal lobes learn associations and patterns through experience with the world. Over time connections between the nerve cells form and stabilise into representations that can support vast stores of **knowledge** (sometimes called '**semantic memory**'; Tulving 1985) about the external world. This store of knowledge not only underpins the capacity that human beings have to understand the world they see, but it also underpins the capacity for **language** by allowing for certain sounds (words) to be mapped onto the different concepts and entities experienced.

Understanding what is seen, and being able to conceptualise and talk about it, depends upon communication between the occipital lobe and temporal lobe, but understanding **how to interact skillfully** with the environment depends instead on communication between the occipital lobe and **parietal lobe**. This region of the cortex is particularly important for **knowing how** to use things. Processing in these networks combines information about visual appearance with bodily information relating to the handling and manipulation of things. This integration of visual and bodily information underpins another important human capability, tool use. An **understanding of space** and of how parts relate to wholes also depends upon the processing that occurs in this region of the brain. The parietal lobe is also vulnerable to damage in dementia, meaning that difficulties with the use and handling of objects (e.g. clothes, household appliances, tools and equipment, knives and forks) frequently appear as symptoms of dementia.

The frontal lobe has a slightly different and higher role within the cortex in that it takes in all the knowledge from the temporal and parietal lobes and uses that knowledge to make decisions about actions and behaviour. The networks of nerve cells in the frontal lobe are vast, even in comparison with those of the temporal and parietal lobes. They provide the processing power necessary to control how knowledge is used through thought and reason to generate plans and goals. Plans and goals are constructed according to the opportunities and threats within the environment. Once a plan has been decided upon, the frontal lobe also has the power to command the body to take action.

Overall, damage to the frontal lobes causes a **dysexecutive syndrome**, meaning problems with the **planning** and **control** functions. However, this is a particularly broad term covering many different component functions. It seems probable that an area as vast as the frontal lobe will be divided such that different parts have different specialisms within the overall goal of providing control and strategy to thought and behaviour. Knowledge about the executive functions of the frontal lobe is still in its infancy, although the upper or lower regions of the frontal lobe appear to have different roles. The upper regions (often called the **dorsolateral** frontal areas) are more involved with the control of the cognitive aspects of thought and reason, whilst the lower regions (often called the **orbitofrontal** areas) are more involved with the control of emotion and social aspects of thought and reason (Fig 1.4).

Figure 1.4   A picture showing the division of the frontal lobe into the dorsolateral and orbitofrontal regions.

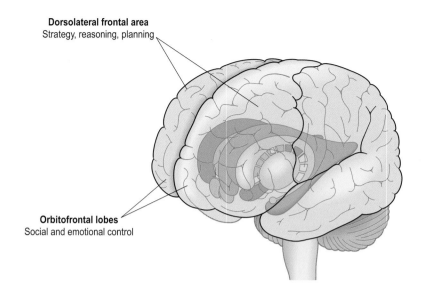

Dorsolateral frontal area
Strategy, reasoning, planning

Orbitofrontal lobes
Social and emotional control

The review above shows that the different lobes of the cerebral cortex have very different functions and sketches out the broad nature of those functions. This next section will focus upon the particular symptoms that a person with dementia is likely to experience should particular lobes be damaged by their condition (as summarised in Table 1.4). It is important to understand that a person can experience some of the difficulties listed in Table 1.4 whilst not having others. You may encounter people who can, for example, use an object successfully but have lost the corresponding knowledge about what it is called or what it is for. This is called a **dissociation**; a serious impairment in one aspect of cognition in combination with retained ability in another. Dissociations are commonly observed following a range of different types of brain damage and also occur in dementia, particularly during the mild to moderate stages where damage may be severe in one lobe, but leave other lobes less affected (Martin et al 1986, Haxby et al 1990). Evidence for dissociations in dementia undermines the old idea that dementia is 'global intellectual decline' as it shows that one aspect of the intellect can be affected independently of other aspects. This is why cognitive profiling is important when working with people with dementia.

Table 1.4 shows that the particular nature of the symptoms to emerge depends firstly upon the lobe that is affected, and secondly upon whether damage is more severe on the left or the right side. We have already seen that the cerebral cortex is divided into **two hemispheres**. Whilst from the outside the two hemispheres look very similar, they are known to have different functions. The **left hemisphere** is particularly important for **language functions** (at least in the majority of people) whilst the **right hemisphere** is more important for **spatial understanding and emotional processing** (reviewed in Kolb & Whishaw 2003). The two sides of the frontal lobe are also likely to have different functions, but due to the complexity of this region the nature of this division of function is less clear. There is

Table 1.4 Summary of symptoms associated with damage to the temporal, parietal and frontal lobes

Cortical area	Function	Symptom
Left temporal lobe	Understanding language Understanding and recognising objects	Anomia/aphasia Agnosia
Right temporal lobe	Understanding and recognising objects Understanding and recognising people	Agnosia Prospoagnosia
Left parietal lobe	Reading Writing Understanding number and calculation Sequencing body movements in skilled action	Alexia Agraphia Acalculia Ideomotor apraxia
Right parietal lobe	Awareness of left side of space Understanding spatial relations and how parts make wholes	Visual neglect Constructional apraxia
Dorsolateral frontal lobe	Control of thought and planning	Dysexecutive syndrome (cognitive)
Orbitofrontal lobe	Control of emotions, instincts and behaviour	Dysexecutive syndrome (social-emotional)

some evidence though, to suggest that the left frontal lobe is important for initiating activities whilst the right frontal lobe is more important for inhibiting or stopping activities. Left frontal lobe damage is also associated with depression, apathy and a lack of interest in other people and life, whilst damage to the right is associated with immature behaviour, agitation, a lack of tact and social graces and coarse or promiscuous behaviour. The symptoms listed in Table 1.4 will now be explained in a little more detail below.

The linguistic nature of the left cerebral hemisphere means that the **left temporal lobe** is especially important for the **mappings between objects and words**. Damage to the left temporal lobe undermines the ability to **understand language**. Words can still be heard, but damage to the networks that can map the words onto their corresponding meanings means that what is heard is often not understood. Damage in this area particularly affects the understanding for content words such as nouns. Grammatical words and constructions are less affected and people with dementia often continue to use the correct grammar but their speech increasingly lacks content as the range of content words available declines (Warrington 1975, Schwartz et al 1979). If the damage is not too severe it may only be the understanding and use of language that is affected and the person may be described as being **aphasic** (a general word for any type of language difficulty) or **anomic** (a specific term for difficulty with naming). If, however, the damage intensifies, or if the damage is more towards the occipital end of the temporal lobe where visual information is coming in, the symptoms may be better considered as an **agnosia** (a word used to describe problems with knowledge and recognition) because the person will have problems understanding what they see as well as what they hear (thus the problem is primarily one of knowledge rather than a specific problem with language).

Equivalent areas in the **right temporal lobe** are thought to support **knowledge of people** and the processes of **face recognition**. Damage to the right temporal lobe can, therefore, cause difficulties in recognising friends and family. These areas have also been found to have a role in understanding the emotional information carried in the tone and prosody of speech. The fact that an understanding of the verbal content of language is dealt with in one side of the brain, whilst an understanding of the emotional intent is dealt with in the other reveals that it must not be assumed that because a person cannot understand the meaning of words they will not understand a harsh or dismissive tone. Furthermore, even if there is damage in the right temporal lobe that affects the analysis of tone of voice, this should not be seen as meaning there is no need to bother about non-verbal communication when interacting with people with dementia. Emotional signals in the tone of voice co-exist with other signals carried in the body. These bodily signals will be picked up by the visual areas of the occipital lobe which, as explained above, are likely to be functioning normally. There are also many subcortical structures that receive information from both the eyes and the ears and perform their own analyses of whether another person is best categorised as friend or foe, albeit below the level of consciousness. **It is extremely important that a loss of knowledge at the highest level is not equated with a total loss of knowledge.** There are deeper levels of knowledge that are more robust in dementia and continue to give people a sense of what is going on, even though they may not be able to articulate or share that knowledge in the usual way (Murdoch et al 1987, Bayles et al 1991, Sabat 2006).

Whilst the right temporal lobe seems to be of particular importance in the emotional functions of the right hemisphere, the **right parietal lobe** plays an important role in the spatial functions associated with this side of the brain. If damage is limited to the right parietal lobe, with no damage in the left, a condition called **visual neglect** can occur in which a person loses awareness of the left side of space. It is, therefore, important to observe people carefully to see whether they ignore events occurring on the left side. Failure to eat the left side of a meal or failure to dress the left side of the body is often a sign of visual neglect. Damage to the right parietal lobe is also associated with problems with **constructional abilities**, that is, problems with understanding the three-dimensional nature of space and problems with building and constructing things. A difficulty with copying drawings, such as the interlocking pentagons from the Mini-Mental State Examination (Folstein et al 1975) is usually an indication of disruption to the right parietal lobe.

The **left parietal lobe** is important for the correct sequencing of body movements during skilled actions. The linguistic nature of the left side means that the ability to write is critically dependent upon this region, as is the ability to read. There is also evidence to connect mathematical abilities to this area. Problems with understanding number (**acalculia**), problems with writing (**agraphia**) and problems with reading (**alexia**) are all associated with left parietal lobe damage and are all common in dementia, although people with mild to moderate Alzheimer's disease often retain the ability to read text out loud, but are not able to understand what they read (Sasanuma et al 1992, Lambon Ralph et al 1995). This pattern suggests a dissociation between temporal lobe function (damaged) and parietal lobe function (intact). The symptoms of alexia, agraphia and acalculia may occur together, or they may occur separately, especially during the mild stages, depending upon where exactly the damage is. However, as a dementia advances it is likely that reading, writing and arithmetic will all be affected and that problems will be accompanied by agnosia (lack of understanding). If agnosia is absent, this would suggest against Alzheimer's disease as the main cause of the dementia. Curiously, damage to the left parietal lobe rarely causes any visual neglect; attention to the right side of space does not seem to be vulnerable to left parietal damage in the same way the attention to the left side of space is vulnerable to damage to the right. The reasons for this are poorly understood.

Turning finally to the frontal lobe, frontotemporal dementia particularly affects the lower, **orbitofrontal regions** of this lobe giving this form of dementia a very characteristic profile in which changes to personality and behaviour dominate over memory loss (Neary & Snowden 2003). The person is likely to become disinhibited and behave in a socially challenging and irresponsible manner that is likely to cause disapproval. A person with orbitofrontal lobe damage has limited ability to control instinctive impulses or to suppress rude comments or thoughts (Damasio 1994). In general, 'ME-NOW' seems to become the prime motivating force. In frontotemporal dementia the changes are dramatic, but similar alterations may occur in all forms of dementia, although usually of less intensity. It is also very important to note that apparent changes in personality can be a normal reaction to an environment which is not responsive to the needs and experiences of the person with dementia, rather than a direct and inevitable consequence of brain damage. This will be explained further in the final section.

Changes in the **dorsolateral regions of the frontal lobe** (see Fig 1.4) affect the ability to plan ahead and to integrate knowledge or verbal instructions into behavioural decisions. There is a good example of the types of problems this can cause for a person with dementia in the Understanding Dementia video produced by the Dementia Services Information and Development Centre (2003), based at St James' Hospital in Dublin. Emily is laying the table with her daughter, but instead of thinking ahead by counting out the number of people having dinner and going to the drawer once to take all the necessary cutlery in one go, Emily becomes involved in what seems like a repetitive and inefficient ritual of going to the drawer, taking a single piece of cutlery out, bringing it to the table and then returning to the drawer to collect the next piece. The daughter points out that it would be quicker to get the cutlery all at once. Emily assents that this is a good plan, and then proceeds with the ritual as before. Emily appears to understand what her daughter says, suggesting that the left temporal lobe is not badly affected, but seems unable to respond to the verbal information. This suggests that her dorsolateral frontal lobe may be damaged, so that even though she understands, the temporal lobe is sending the information up to a frontal lobe network that can no longer integrate the knowledge into her decisions and behaviour.

The behaviour of people with frontal lobe damage, therefore, becomes very sensitive to the environment. Certain things we see or hear automatically stimulate certain responses. Within the kitchen environment, Emily retains enough ability to know that the drawer should be opened, the fork taken out and taken to the table, but she has lost the 'bigger picture' element that allows her to think about the whole activity she is undertaking and use either her own knowledge or instruction from others to generate the higher level plan that could make her behaviour more efficient. The lessons to be learnt from this are, first, we should not become frustrated if instructions seem to be understood and then ignored. This is likely to reflect brain damage rather than a desire to be difficult and obtuse. And, second, that in understanding the behaviour of people with dementia, we need to be very aware of what is in the environment and the habits and instincts that objects or people may stimulate. This is important when assessing activities of daily living because assessment in the unusual environment of the out-patient clinic may indicate a higher level of disability than assessment within the normal home environment.

Another reason to be very aware of the environment when assessing the behaviour of people with dementia relates to the dual function of the frontal lobe as both initiator and inhibitor. This can lead to an apparently paradoxical situation in which a person can be apathetic at some times and restless or disinhibited at others. Careful observation of the environment may reveal that certain stimuli or situations trigger responses or habits the person may have difficulty stopping (e.g. opening and shutting doors, manipulating objects), whilst at other times a lack of stimulation or change may result in the person having difficulty starting activities and becoming apathetic. Brain function is also affected by the circadian rhythm (natural alterations in alertness that happen during the course of 24 hours) so where a person is experiencing either apathy or restlessness it is also important to look for patterns related to the time of day.

This concludes the basic review of the cerebral cortex and how its functions are divided over its vast surface area into the four lobes. It is hoped you now have a good understanding of where the symptoms of dementia come from, and also of why there is considerable variation from one person to the next in terms of the particular symptoms they experience. This provides the foundation from which we can begin to understand the complex interplay between brain damage and the factors highlighted by Kitwood (1997). It is important to go beyond this simple mapping of symptoms onto the surface of the brain and consider what damage to the cortex means in terms of the lived experience of the person with dementia. A human life involves many varied and rich experiences. These experiences determine the patterns of connections that form within the networks of the cortex. Thus, whilst every person has a cortex and the key function of that cortex is to learn, exactly what is learnt and represented within that cortex will be unique to that individual. The patterns of connections within a person's cortex are as individual as their fingerprint, and also far more powerful in determining their individuality and identity. Much of the cortex, particularly in the temporal lobe, is dedicated to learning from experience and representing the experiences of our life. The function of memory, and how damage to the systems that support memory fundamentally alters a person's lived experience of the world, will be reviewed in the final section.

MEMORY

In the review of the higher cognitive functions supported by the cerebral cortex, memory has not been discussed. Memory is a very complex function of the brain and is particularly vulnerable to dementia, especially Alzheimer's disease. The human ability to be able to remember complex events from life depends upon complex interactions between the cerebral cortex and a subcortical structure just below the cerebral cortex of the temporal lobe called the hippocampus. Figure 1.5 shows the inside surface of the right cerebral hemisphere. You can see that the cortex of the frontal, parietal and occipital lobes continues on this inner surface whilst the hippocampus is found on the inner surface of the temporal lobe. (Although it is common practice to talk about 'the hippocampus' we actually have two of them – one in the right hemisphere and one in the left.) We have already seen that the networks of nerve cells in the temporal and parietal lobes of the cortex provide knowledge networks that allow for a detailed understanding of the world and how to interact with that world. The knowledge in the temporal and parietal regions of the cortex builds up slowly. It takes many repeated experiences with things for the required representations

Figure 1.5   A picture showing the inner surface of the right hemisphere and the location of the hippocampus and amygdala.

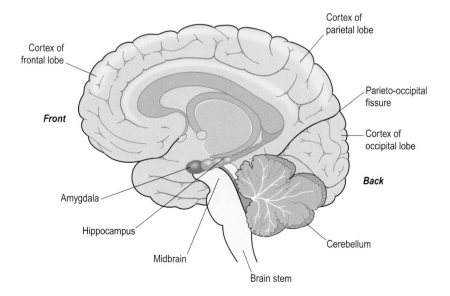

to form and so these areas are ideal for supporting knowledge of truths about the world which undergo little or slow change. Human beings, however, also have the ability to remember specific events and experiences from their lives following a single experience, and this is due to the ability of the hippocampus to tie many different aspects of an experience together into a single representation that underpins the memory for that experience. This type of memory is sometimes called **'episodic memory'** (Tulving 1985).

There are complex interactions between the episodic memory networks of the hippocampus and the **semantic memory** networks of the temporal lobe. When a person experiences a memory about their life, the hippocampus calls upon the cerebral cortex to 'replay' the experience. Thus, the original pattern of activation across all the different sensory and knowledge areas of the cerebral cortex that were activated during experience of the original event are re-activated, although usually in a muted and fragmented form, explaining why memories lack detail and vividness relative to the original experience. Some important memories get 'replayed' many times through our lives, meaning that the connections between the different cortical areas involved in representing that memory become strengthened and that memory comes to have a separate representation within the semantic memory networks of the temporal lobe as well as within the episodic memory networks of the hippocampus. There are theories that one purpose of dreaming is to consolidate important memories within the semantic memory networks through intense replay of daily experiences (McClelland et al 1995).

The hippocampus is especially vulnerable to Alzheimer's disease. The pathology first takes hold in this structure, later spreading out to affect the cerebral cortex. By the time the symptoms are severe enough for dementia to be diagnosed, the hippocampus is severely depleted of cells and episodic memory function is almost entirely lost (Weingartner et al 1981, Braak & Braak 1991, Welsh et al 1992, Hodges 1998). The loss of the hippocampus undermines the ability to form new memories with respect to ongoing experience. This explains why people with Alzheimer's disease often retain memories from the distant past but have great difficulty in remembering recent events. Recent memory, however, is hit on two fronts when the pathology spreads out to affect the cerebral cortex because as the pathology begins to spread outwards from the hippocampal regions, the semantic memory networks of the temporal lobe are usually the next focus of attack (Van Hoesen & Damasio 1987, Braak & Braak 1991). When these networks begin to fall apart, memories represented within the semantic memory networks also become vulnerable. However, because the oldest memories tend to be those with the strongest representations the networks operate on a 'last in, first out' basis. The semantic memory base of the person with Alzheimer's disease, therefore, tends to drift increasingly into the past as the disease advances. The combined damage to both episodic and semantic memory makes it increasingly difficult for the present to gain any foothold within the person's conscious understanding of the world.

It is important to understand that memory is rarely experienced as a passive mental state, but is usually at the heart of active processes involving communication between many different brain structures. Memory functions, therefore, are more actively involved in other cognitive functions (e.g. perception, decision-making) than is commonly realised. The knowledge base of semantic memory interprets current perceptions to provide understanding of the things seen in the 'here and now'. For the person with advancing Alzheimer's disease, the store of information available for interpreting the here and now becomes dominated by events of long ago. The brain will, however, continue to use whatever information is available to make sense of what is happening now. This helps to explain why people with dementia can have difficulty in interpreting their current environment and their role within it. If a person is moved to a residential home, for example, the person may no longer have the full brain circuitry required to form new memories that would explain that move and allow them to understand where this is and why they are here. Even if the person is living at home, memories of their childhood home may rise to the fore, meaning they do not feel they are at home and are restless to get back to a home of long ago.

The representations and beliefs generated in the memory systems of the temporal lobe also feed forward into the decision-making networks of the frontal lobe, and downwards to influence the operation of all the underlying structures. Understanding changes to the internal belief states of people with dementia is, therefore, fundamental to understanding their behaviour. Imagine, for example, a woman with dementia who believes she is the mother of small children, as she was 40 years ago. She may notice that her children are not with her and become very anxious. If she believes she has lost her children, she will behave like a mother who has lost her children. She might start a frantic search, screaming the name of her child. People who do not understand the nature of her neurological impairment are likely to dismiss such behaviour as disruptive and unnecessary. Such behaviour is likely to be seen as being symptomatic of dementia and primarily attributable to brain damage. However, whilst brain damage has played its part in altering her internal reality, the behaviour is more complex, resulting from an interaction between her environment (which lacks her child) and her brain damage (which makes her believe he/she should be there).

In assessing the impact of the environment upon the behaviour of a person with dementia it is important to be aware of the functions of another structure that lies underneath the cortex called the **amygdala** (see Fig 1.5). Amygdala means almond, and it is a small almond shape structure that sits directly in front of the hippocampus (as with the hippocampus, although it is common to talk of 'the amygdala' there are two of these, one in the right and one in the left). The amygdala is at the centre of the brain's emotional processes, and is particularly important in mediating negative emotions such as anger and fear, including the defensive behaviours associated with these emotions. The amygdala has direct links with the autonomic nervous system, which has two branches, the **sympathetic 'fight or flight' branch** and the **parasympathetic 'rest and digest' branch**. If the amygdala picks up any hint of a threat in the external environment it immediately activates the 'fight or flight' branch so that the body is prepared to take defensive action. If a person with dementia enters an unfamiliar and complex environment (such as a hospital, day centre or residential home) the unfamiliar and complex nature of the place is likely to stimulate the amygdala, resulting in threat-related emotions and behaviours. Again, this is a normal response to a challenging environment rather than a sign of deterioration and further brain damage. How would you feel if you were suddenly taken to the centre of Tokyo and left there without a guidebook?

It is common for people without dementia to feel that people with dementia should continue to conform to the dictates of 'our reality' and to become frustrated when people with dementia are unable to conform. People with dementia are often labelled as being manipulative, deliberately difficult or attention seeking when they are unable to conform to expectations. However, the failure of understanding here lies more with the people without dementia than the people with dementia. Instead of analysing the environment to identify threat signals which, as people without dementia, they are blind to, people without dementia often intensify the distress by not taking the beliefs of the person with dementia seriously. Imagine you lost your child in ASDA and when you went to the staff to ask for help they explained that you could not really have a child because you are too old and should sit down and have a cup of tea until you felt better. How would you react? Would you gratefully accept the cup of tea or would you become very angry, perhaps even aggressive, because they would not believe that you had lost your child?

The behaviour of other people is especially important in determining whether people with dementia feel threatened by their environment or safe within it. It is vitally important that everything possible is done to make both the physical and social environment supportive rather than frightening for people with dementia. Once a person has a diagnosis of dementia they are likely to be brought into contact with a huge number of different professionals and support workers. Problems with perception and memory make it very difficult to remember and understand who is who or to know whether a particular person means them ill or good. The amygdala is highly sensitive to the signals carried in body language as to whether another human being is more likely to be friend or foe. Thus, how those professionals and support workers behave is critical in determining whether the person's amygdala will be stimulating 'fight or flight' or 'rest and digest' emotions and behaviours.

Indeed, it is very easy to map many of the so-called 'behavioural symptoms of dementia' onto the normal defensive responses organised by the amygdala, as shown in Table 1.5.

Retention of lower structures in the hierarchy of the brain, together with the fact the cortex is only partially rather than wholly damaged, means that the brain of a person with dementia continues to try to do its basic job, of regulating behaviour and activity to meet the needs and desires of its owner. Damage to the cortex affects the person's detailed understanding and awareness of the world about them and is likely to affect their belief system such that they are no longer able to understand and respond to the dictates of 'our reality'. However, whilst their brain might be damaged it is nonetheless their brain, and not the brain of a cognitively intact other, that controls their behaviour. The capacity for sensation and action is not lost, just the understanding part in between. The areas of the cortex that

Table 1.5 Symptoms of dementia or normal responses to frightening and unsupportive situations?

Fight	Aggression
	Anger
Flight	Anxiety
	Desire to escape
Flock	Following
	Attachment behaviours
Freeze	Apathy
	Withdrawal

Table 1.6 Safe signals for positive emotion

Objects/photographs that are familiar and comforting

Environment that is pleasant, calm and simple (but not cold and clinical)

People whose genuine commitment to the person with dementia is apparent in both their verbal and non-verbal behaviours

Suitable activity

Needs and beliefs understood, acknowledged and responded to

support feelings and consciousness are not usually damaged, so it does not follow that because a person has lost memory and cognitive ability they have lost the capacity to feel negative emotions, such as pain and fear, or positive emotions such as interest and happiness.

Dementia care, therefore, has to be much more than simply keeping people alive. It is essential to attend to the person's continued sense of existing as a particular person, with beliefs and needs and feelings just like anyone else. People with dementia experience states of ill-being and of wellbeing. Promotion of wellbeing amongst people with dementia depends upon them living in an environment that sends messages of safety and not messages of threat or neglect. People with dementia retain enough brain power to know whether they are being treated as a 'PERSON with dementia', or a 'person with DEMENTIA' and they will feel and behave accordingly. Table 1.6 summarises some of the measures that can be taken to allow people with dementia to feel safe despite the challenging nature of the condition they live with.

CONCLUSION

This chapter has provided a review of recent knowledge about dementia and the brain. It should help you to understand what dementia is and to understand the nature of the challenges faced by people with living with primary dementia. The review of the brain shows that dementia is focused within a particular part of the brain, the cerebral cortex. This is a vast and powerful structure and the particular symptoms a person experiences depends upon where exactly it is damaged. This knowledge should help you to understand the most common symptoms of dementia and where they come from. More importantly, however, the review has gone beyond the simple mapping of symptoms to explain what it might be like to live inside the world of someone whose cortex has been damaged, particularly someone whose memory system has been altered so that representations and beliefs about the past dominate over those relating to the present. Moving inside the brain of the person with dementia helps to understand behaviours which might otherwise be viewed as being deviant and disruptive and places the role of brain damage within its proper context.

Difficult or disruptive behaviours are not attributable solely to brain damage and it is important this is understood as such attributions encourage the belief that nothing can be done to help people with dementia and pushes management in the direction of stopping or containing the behaviours (often through drugs or physical restraint) rather than looking deeper into the complex causes of the behaviours and the feelings of ill-being that accompany them. In reality, the person's physical and social environment is likely to be of equal importance in driving such behaviours and might also be open to easy modifications which would promote the person's wellbeing, and so reduce the behaviours. This chapter has provided the foundations upon which we can see why it is important to recognise the personhood and experiences of people with dementia and focus care on promoting their wellbeing, rather than managing and containing their symptoms. The remainder of this book reveals the methods and techniques that can be used to achieve this goal.

References

Audit Commission 2002 Forget Me Not 2002 Developing mental health services for older people in England. Audit Commission, London

Ballard C, Bannister C 2005 Criteria for the diagnosis of dementia. In: Burns A, O'Brien J, Ames D (eds) Dementia. Hodder-Arnold, London, p 24–37

Bayles KA, Tomoeda CK, Kaszniak A, Trosset MW 1991 Alzheimer's disease effects on semantic memory: loss of structure or impaired processing? Journal of Cognitive Neuroscience 3:166–182

Braak H, Braak E 1991 Neuropathological staging of Alzheimer-related changes. Acta Neuropathologica (Berlin) 82:239–259

Brooker D 2007 Person-centred dementia care: making services better. Jessica Kingsley, London.

Chui HC, Victoroff JJ, Margolin D, Jagust W, Shankle R, Katzman R 1992 Criteria for the diagnosis of ischaemic vascular dementia proposed by the State of California Alzheimer's Disease Diagnostic and Treatment Centers. Neurology 42:473–480

Corey-Bloom J, Fleisher A 2005 The natural history of Alzheimer's disease. In: Burns A, O'Brien J, Ames D (eds) Dementia. Hodder-Arnold, London, p 376–386

Damasio AR 1994 Descartes' error. Papermac, London

Dementia Services Information and Development Centre 2003 Understanding dementia (DVD). Milbrook Studios, Dublin.

Department of Health 2001 National service framework for older people. Department of Health (DoH), London

Downs MG 1996 The role of general practice and the primary care team in dementia diagnosis and management. International Journal of Geriatric Psychiatry 11:937–942

Downs MG, Clibbens R, Rae C, Cook A, Woods R 2002 What do general practitioners tell people with dementia and their families about their condition? Dementia 1:47–58

Drickamer M, Lachs M 1992 Should patients with Alzheimer's disease be told their diagnosis? New England Journal of Medicine 326:947–951

Esiri MM, Matthews F, Brayne C et al 2001 Pathological correlates of late-onset dementia in a multicentre, community-based population in England and Wales. Lancet 357:169–175

Folstein MF, Folstein SE, McHugh PR 1975 "Mini mental state": A practical method for grading the cognitive state of patients for the clinician. Journal of Psychiatric Research 12(3):189–198

Haxby JV, Grady CL, Koss E et al 1990 Longitudinal study of cerebral metabolic asymmetries and associated neuropsychological patterns in early dementia of the Alzheimer type. Archives of Neurology 47:753–760

Hodges JR 1998 The amnestic prodrome of Alzheimer's disease. Brain 121:1601–1602

Kitwood T 1989 Brain, mind and dementia: with particular reference to Alzheimer's disease. Ageing and Society 9:1–15

Kitwood T 1997 Dementia reconsidered. Open University Press, Buckingham.

Kolb B, Whishaw IQ 2003 Fundamentals of human neuropsychology, 5th edn. Worth Publishers, New York, p 414–417

Lambon Ralph MA, Ellis AW, Franklin S 1995 Semantic loss without surface dyslexia. Neurocase 1:363–369

The Lund and Manchester Groups 1994 Clinical and neuropathological criteria for frontotemporal dementia. Journal of Neurology, Neurosurgery and Psychiatry 57:416–418

McClelland JL, McNaughton B, O'Reilly RC 1995 Why there are complementary learning systems in the hippocampus and neocortex: insights from the successes and failures of connectionist models of learning and memory. Psychological Review 102:419–457

McKeith IG, Galasko D, Kosaka K et al 1996 Consensus guidelines for the clinical and pathologic diagnosis of dementia with Lewy bodies (DLB): report of the consortium on DLB international workshop. Neurology 47:1113–1124

McKhann G, Drachman D, Folstein M, Katzman R, Price D, Stadlan EM 1984 Clinical diagnosis of Alzheimer's disease: report of the NINCDS-ADRDA Work Group under the auspices of Department of Health and Human Services Task Force on Alzheimer's Disease. Neurology 34:939–944

Martin A, Brouwers P, Lalonde F, Cox C, Teleska P, Fedio P 1986 Towards a behavioural typology of Alzheimer's patients. Journal of Clinical and Experimental Neuropsychology 8:594–610

Meyers BS 1997 Telling patients they have Alzheimer's disease: Important for planning their future and no evidence of ill effects. British Medical Journal 314:321–332

Murdoch BE, Chenery HJ, Wilks V, Boyle RS 1987 Language disorders in dementia of the Alzheimer type. Brain and Language 31:122–137

National Audit Office 2007 Improving services and support for people with dementia. London, The Stationery Office

National Institute for Clinical Excellence 2006a Dementia: supporting people with dementia and their carers in health and social care. NICE, London

National Institute for Clinical Excellence 2006b Donepezil, galantamine, rivastigmine (review) and memantine for the treatment of Alzheimer's disease. NICE, London

Neary D, Snowden J 2003 Causes of dementia in younger people. In: Baldwin R, Murray M (eds) Younger people with dementia: a multidisciplinary approach. Martin Dunitz, London, p 7–41

O'Brien JT 2006 NICE and anti-dementia drugs: a triumph of health economics over clinical wisdom? The Lancet Neurology 5:994–996

Renshaw J, Scurfield P, Cloke L, Orrell M 2001 General practitioners' views on the early diagnosis of dementia. British Journal of General Practice 51:37–38

Rogers CR 1961 On becoming a person. Houghton Mifflin, Boston MA

Roman GC, Tatemichi TK, Erkinjuntii T 1993 Vascular dementia: diagnostic criteria for research studies. Report of the NINDS-AIREN International Workshop. Neurology 43:250–260

Sabat SR 2006 Implicit memory and people with Alzheimer's disease: implications for care giving. American Journal of Alzheimer's Disease and Other Disorders 21:11–14

Sasanuma S, Sakuma N, Kitano K 1992 Reading kanji without semantics: evidence from a longitudinal study of dementia. Cognitive Neuropsychology 9:465–486

Schwartz MF, Marin OSM, Saffran EM 1979 Dissociations of language function in dementia: a case study. Brain and Language 7:277–306

Takeda A, Loveman E, Clegg A 2006 A systematic review of the clinical effectiveness of donepezil, rivastigmine and galantamine on cognition, quality of life and adverse events in Alzheimer's disease. International Journal of Geriatric Psychiatry 21:17–28

Tulving E 1985 How many memory systems are there? American Psychologist 40:385–398

Van Hoesen GW, Damasio AR 1987 Neural correlates of cognitive impairment in Alzheimer's disease. In: Mountcastle VB, Plum F, Oeiger SR (eds) Handbook of physiology, Volume 5. American Physiological Society, Bethesda

Vassilas CA, Donaldson J 1998 Telling the truth: what do general practitioners say to people with dementia or terminal cancer? British Journal of General Practice 48:1081–1082

Warrington EK 1975 The selective impairment of semantic memory. Quarterly Journal of Experimental Psychology 27:635–657

Weingartner H, Kaye W, Smallberg SA, Eberg MH, Gillin JC, Sitaram N 1981 Memory failures in progressive idiopathic dementia. Journal of Abnormal Psychology 90:187–196

Welsh KA, Butters N, Hughes JP, Mohs RC, Heyman A 1992 Detection and staging of dementia in Alzheimer's disease: use of neuropsychological measures developed for the Consortium to Establish a Registry for Alzheimer's Disease (CERAD). Archives of Neurology 49:448–452

Whalley L 2001 The ageing brain. Phoenix, London

World Health Organization 1993 ICD-10 Classification of Mental and Behavioural Disorders. Diagnostic Criteria for Research. World Health Organization, Geneva

Chapter 2

Occupational therapy revisited

INTRODUCTION

Perhaps the most serious challenge that our profession and our educational systems have had to deal with in recent years has been the diversity of practice that comes under the occupational therapy umbrella. A fly on the wall who didn't know any better would look at a therapist using drama with people who have learning difficulties, and at another engaged in dressing practice on a stroke unit, and know for sure that these two people were from different professions. For whilst of course there is a common base in occupation, there is little resemblance in the day-to-day professional practice of the two. Such is the richness of occupational life, and the diversity of occupational need.

Since the early days of the profession, both in general and mental health settings, an understanding of the role of occupation in health and wellbeing has increased and spread, as has a concurrent demand for occupational therapy and occupational therapists in all kinds of disability contexts. Practice, it seems though, has rushed ahead of theory, and whilst we are still engaging in debate about the profession's core values and comparing this model with that, community pressure demands action – in terminal care, in family therapy, in forensic psychiatry, in environmental design, etc. These are all areas of health care (and there are many more examples) in which occupational therapy is a relative newcomer. Dementia care is another.

Occupational therapy began to make its presence felt in dementia care during the late 1970s and 1980s with the creation of the first posts for occupational therapists in the context of residential and nursing homes. We might say that it has been perhaps around 30 years in its development so far. In those early years there was little in the way of a theory base to underpin practice and the concept of models was still (in the UK at least) in its infancy. Those of us attracted to work in the dementia care field found ourselves struggling with an existing philosophy which didn't 'fit' with the problems we were experiencing in clinical practice.

The predominant value base of the time prized above all things independence, mastery, autonomy; the individuals should learn or relearn to 'do' for himself. Models were developing around concepts of adaptation, rehabilitation and self-actualisation, and many of us became entangled in trying to meet the problems of dementia with a frame of reference centred around notions of functional independence. We found ourselves trying to fit the person to the theory, effectively to deal with the practical problems of degeneration by recourse to theories of regeneration. It didn't work, and led us into very real ethical and practical difficulties.

The conflict we had was illustrated neatly and rather picturesquely at the time by a paper which asked us the question, 'Does it matter whether it's Tuesday or Friday?' (Morton & Bleathman 1988). This article was actually written to promote a validation approach to therapy over reality orientation. It is a matter which would not generate a great deal of interest today, nevertheless the core of the argument (wellbeing or independence as the priority for intervention) continues 20 years on. It raised an issue of considerable significance for the occupational therapist, for in the tradition of occupational therapy, it is the task of the occupational therapist to find ways of ensuring that Mrs Bloggs does know the difference between Tuesday and Friday. Cognitive and daily living functions are at stake here, for if she doesn't remember that Tuesday and Friday are her day centre days or daughter-visiting days or whatever, her functional independence in the real world is impaired. (It can also be extremely irritating for the day centre driver and the daughter.) But Morton & Bleathman were arguing that a practice-centred approach (reality orientation is the treatment for memory disorder), which fails to understand the over-riding needs of the person in question, not only misses the mark of therapy, but can actually be damaging and counter-productive.

What is important to Mrs Bloggs? She may of course have some insight into her memory deficit, and request and appreciate help in this matter. But are we sure about that? Why do we feel constrained to have her tackle this memory problem? Is it a request from relatives? Is it because day care staff get very tetchy about wasted journeys and empty places? Is it because we have an ingrained need to return aberrant behaviour to conformity? Or is it simply that we are driven by the whole ethos of our profession, which insists that therapy returns somebody from the sickness or disability they have suffered, to the person they were before (or as near as possible). We believe that such an approach has in many instances been detrimental, and sometimes even damaging to the person it was intended to help. Will it help Mrs Bloggs to have constant reminders of her memory deficit? Does she welcome environmental aids? Is she happy about attending a centre where there will be people who will portray what she might become? Does it really matter whether it's Tuesday or Friday? That is the critical question every practitioner must ask as he or she approaches a new client – is striving to return or to improve function the first priority? If it is, existing models of intervention will suffice. If it isn't, there has to be an alternative; there is little accommodation in a model of rehabilitation for the problems of a degenerative condition.

It is the purpose of this text to propose an alternative, and in the ensuing chapters we offer what is perhaps a basic framework or a matrix from which to develop effective and skilful interventions. It is our hope that if such a framework finds a resonance with other practitioners in dementia care, it will be subjected to consideration and debate, modification and development, in the tradition of most practice tools. It is not our intention that it should be perceived as a definitive model for dementia care; it simply represents our thinking on the matter to date.

We have in the preceding paragraphs posed a challenge to the adequacy of the existing basic paradigm of occupational therapy to accommodate a degenerative condition such as dementia. Such a challenge is not simply a call for a new model, but actually reverberates down through the very ethos of our professional existence. If we are going to propose something different, we need to return to roots. In the rest of this chapter we propose to look again at the nature of occupation and its relation to health, and we want particularly to address the issues of meaning and creativity in health. We conclude by suggesting an alternative focus for occupational therapy in dementia care.

OCCUPATION

Along with models and frames of reference, terminological definitions have generated much discussion over the years. For the purists, definitions of occupation and activity were recently agreed by the European Network of Occupational Therapy in Higher Education (2006; http://www.enothe.hva.nl/). Whilst we don't have a problem with the accuracy of these definitions, we find them bland and not very helpful for our purposes. We have preferred to squeeze out some of the etymological richness of the words by looking at their roots.

We need first perhaps, to say something about the ubiquitous use of the word 'activity' as a term synonymous with occupation. The interchange of these terms may not occur amongst therapists, but it certainly does in dementia care settings generally, where people are unused to the concept of occupation. Mary Reilly (1962) was the first to point out that:

'the major crisis in the proof of our hypothesis (that man, through the use of his hands as they are energised by mind and will, may influence the state of his own health) will ... be ... to know the difference between activity and occupation, and to act on the knowledge of this difference.'

A few minutes in the company of a good dictionary is sufficient to introduce us to that difference. The word activity very simply (and rather vaguely) means 'a thing done', and to act is 'to do a thing'. The word occupation, however, is multifaceted, having a broad variation in shades of meaning. There are in fact some seven different core meanings, which can be summarised as follows:

- the seizing or taking possession of (by force) – as an army invading a land
- a holding – as a place or piece of land held by a tenant
- the taking or filling up (of time or space)
- that in which one is engaged (person, mind, attention)
- action in which one is engaged habitually
- the investment of money or capital in
- the dwelling or residing in.

We might suggest then, if we weave together these seven facets of meaning, that we have a composite which is of considerable utility for our purposes. *Occupation is that which we seize for our own personal possession, and which, because it holds meaning and value for us, habitually and fully engages our time, attention and environment.* This interpretation, stopping short as it does of any specification as to what 'that' might be, is of considerable import as a cornerstone of our discussion. The very non-specificity of the concept is, and has been, both the joy and the frustration, the freedom and the constraint, the goad and the halter of our professional progress. In one sense it is of course not the business of occupational therapy (or any other therapy) to dictate what 'that' is. 'That' is something inherently subjective; it is something that ultimately each person for himself must decide.

This subjectivity presents a two-fold challenge to the therapist. On the one hand it militates against prescriptive practice, demanding a fully person-centred and person-led approach to therapeutic intervention. On the other, it presents major difficulties to the profession's framing of the service it has to offer. How can a profession set its parameters for practice, when the core problem (occupational dysfunction) is so infinitely diverse across humankind? This has been a major dilemma over at least four decades; a dilemma which led to an almost complete derailment of the profession during the 1970s, bringing not inconsiderable anguish to those of us engaged in the conflict. Times, and professional development have moved on since then, and we do now have a rich body of knowledge at the core of our theoretical structure. Nevertheless, judging by the continuing debate in the literature, we have still not yet achieved a full congruence and coherence of theory which satisfies the thoughtful practitioner. We are still, in Hagedorn's (1995) terms 'in search of the core'. It is not within the remit of this text (or the gift of the authors) to address this wider issue, but it may be that abler brains in the future will perceive our proposed view in the broader perspective of professional development. We hope so.

For the purposes of this text, we take as our main underpinning premise the definition of occupation suggested above, and we shall return to it from time to time in the course of the ensuing discussion.

OCCUPATION AND WELLNESS

In our context of dementia care, we need to look again at what we mean by health, and at its focus in our professional practice. Health is actually considerably more difficult to define than occupation. There can in fact be no universal declaration on the nature of health for the reason of its very subjectivity; that which is health to one person, is not to another. The World Health Organization, however, constrained by its constitution to attempt such, stated in 1947 that:

'Health is a state of complete physical, mental and social wellbeing, and is not merely the absence of disease or infirmity.'

Occupational therapist Johnson (1986) has suggested something similar:

'Integrity of body, mind, spirit and emotions that is available in the presence or absence of illness, disease or disability.'

Black's Medical Dictionary describes health as:

'... the highest state of mental and bodily vigour of which any given individual is capable.'

All these offerings refer to a state, a condition which by definition is absolute, a 'position achieved' as it were. However, the biologist Dubos (1980) is critical of such definitions, describing the concept of a state of perfect health as a mirage, 'a utopian creation of the human mind'. He suggests that the concept cannot become a reality, because the often hostile and ever-changing nature of the human environment will always ensure that such a peak of adaptation is never achieved. Gordon (1958), a medical officer of health, is of a similar mind:

'To maintain his equilibrium with his environment, man and his species are in perpetual struggle – with microbes, with incompatible mothers-in-law, with drunken car drivers, and with cosmic rays from Outer Space. How then in this context of movement and buffeting back and forth between organism and environment, can we find any place for the woolly-headed definitions of "positive health", as a state that can and must be considered apart from disease?'

Wellness (a term coined only a few years ago), in contrast to health, seems to be something rather subtly different; a concept which has a rather more dynamic quality about it. Indeed Opatz (1985) has described wellness not as a state but as a process: 'the process of adapting patterns of behaviour'. This notion is supported by Berry & Berry (1984), who suggest that wellness is a process of creating awareness, motivating, fostering attitudes and actions, towards the goal of functioning at optimum level. They employ a picturesque, if somewhat ungrammatical, metaphor in clarification:

'Wellness could be described as a mountain riddled with deep gorges, giant boulders, and dense forests that must be climbed.'

This notion of an effortful *striving in action*, is a thread that is woven through the ideas of a number of commentators on health and disease, who reject the idea of homeostasis as synonymous with health. Indeed the message seems to be that tension (or the right amount of tension) *is* health.

> 'The "positiveness" of health does not lie in the state, but in the struggle – the effort to reach a goal which in its perfection is unattainable.' (Gordon 1958)

Webster's dictionary defines tension as a (dynamic) balance between two opposing forces, a helpful concept for the purposes of this discussion. We might thereby see the person in wellness as being the person who is achieving a balance, that 'balance' actually being a striving in action: a process not a state.

> '... mental health is based on a certain degree of tension, the tension between what one has already achieved and what one still ought to accomplish, or the gap between what one is and what one ought to become ... I consider it a dangerous misconception of mental hygiene to assume that what man needs is equilibrium or, as it is called in biology, "homeostasis" i.e. a tension-less state. What man actually needs is not a tensionless state but rather the striving and struggling for some goal worthy of him.' (Frankl 1963)

Implicit in this idea of wellness as a striving in action are issues relating to personal responsibility for health and wellbeing: healing from within rather than from without. Illich (1975) has noted how the 'epidemic of modern medicine' has removed from the vast majority of humankind any real sense of personal responsibility for their own wellness, and has fostered a debilitating dependence and a misperception of drugs and surgery as the cure for all ills. Naisbitt (1982) has underscored this contention, affirming society's increasing trend over the last decade or so, away from that dependence towards a position of at least a degree of personal responsibility. His discussion on 'institutional help to self-help' charts the self-help and group support mechanisms that have flourished increasingly in the western world in latter years. Capra (1982) too, maintains that health care of the future will mean people taking care of their own health individually and as a society.

Returning to Berry & Berry's mountain image then, we might propose that wellness is not a passive ease, nor comfort, nor contentment, but rather a climb, an engaging with the obstacle, an exertion, a striving, an overcoming. There are places of rest, oases of calm, pinnacles from which the view is magnificent, but the journey is always onward and upward. There are guides and companions, but nobody to offer a piggy-back; the effort is the climber's alone.

The journalist Norman Cousins (1979) in his account of personal illness and recovery, offers a graphic picture of that striving in action. Cousins was smitten in mid-life with an acute onset collagen disease, which in the course of time was diagnosed as ankylosing spondylitis. This is an arthritic condition which is characterised by a gradual fusion of the proximal joints of the body, notably the spine, which ultimately lose all flexibility. Cousins was seriously ill in the acute stages, and was offered a 1 in 500 chance of recovery. Very unhappy about the quality of hospital treatment he was receiving, he decided that he needed to take the responsibility for his own healing into his own hands, and this he did with the assistance of a sympathetic general practitioner. In terms of a striving in action, it was clear that Cousins had no problems about the *striving*: 'there was nothing undersized about my will to live.' The *action* part was more difficult, as he was bed-bound, and almost completely rigid throughout all his joints.

What he decided he must do, was to laugh. Cousins was aware of the psychosomatic effects of positive and negative emotion, and believed that actively pursuing positive emotions would impact upon his body with some kind of a restorative function. To this end he started to watch comic films, and have read to him humorous books. He found that 10 minutes genuine laughter would earn him 2 hours respite from pain. More objectively, his erythrocyte sedimentation rate (ESR) was measured before and after each laughter session. The ESR is a common diagnostic test which indicates severity of inflammation or infection. After each laughter session his ESR had dropped by five points, and this effect was found to be cumulative. As an adjunct to his laughter therapy, Cousins and his physician experimented with massive doses of ascorbic acid (vitamin C); this also was found to reduce his ESR dramatically. Recovery was gradual over months and years, but at the time of writing, Cousins was pain-free and sufficiently mobile to play tennis and ride a horse. He gives much credit for his recovery to the ascorbic acid regime, but is unequivocal in his assertion that personal responsibility for wellness is critical. He believes hospital cultures to be iatrogenic, and that a major feature of his own recovery lay in his removal from hospital and a working partnership with a wise physician.

> '*Dr Hitzig was willing to set aside the large armamentarium of powerful drugs available to the modern physician* when he became convinced that his patient might have something better to offer.' *(Cousins 1979 – ours)*

It is the notion of tension, of striving in action, that we want to hang on to as we continue our discussion into an exploration of meaning, or the place of meaning in occupation and occupational therapy.

OCCUPATION AND MEANING

Engelhardt (1983) has made the rather lofty assertion that occupational therapists are, or should be, custodians of meaning – at least in the context of adaptation to disability. This is a grandiose and rather self-important notion to be sure, but nevertheless one that has some substance given the history and tradition of occupational therapy. From the early exponents of occupation as therapy until the present time, there has been a more or less tacit understanding that therapists' concern with the occupational identity of individuals predicates a concern with the apprehension of meaning(s) in life. Thus it is an underpinning tenet of occupational therapy that for a person to engage in occupation, as opposed merely to doing an activity, the occupation must hold meaning for them; and this is as true for the person in health and wellbeing, as it is for the person in sickness or disability.

The concept of meaning in life is an elusive one, and if occupational therapists are indeed potential custodians of meaning, then they have done precious little to extend the profession's understanding of its function in health and adaptation. This is rather surprising in view of the fact that apprehension of meaning lies at the core of human existence; but maybe the reason for the profession's negligence in this area lies in the pragmatic (as opposed to the philosophical) tradition of occupational therapy and therapists.

Some commentators suggest that meaning can only logically be understood in the context of purpose, that the two phenomena are tightly intermeshed. Occupational therapist Sharrott (1983) maintains that an action is meaningful if it serves a practical purpose, the purpose or goal of an action giving meaning to those steps taken to achieve that goal – purpose becomes the context for meaning.

The Austrian psychotherapist Viktor Frankl, from his concentration camp experiences, is well qualified to discuss the nature of meaning. In essence, his writings support the above view. Frankl (1963) contends that meaning in life may be discovered through what we give to life in terms of our creative works, through what we take from the world in terms of our experiencing values, and through suffering, as the stand we take towards a fate we can no longer change. Thus, Frankl asserts that meaning might be discovered in any of the vicissitudes of life, even in situations where people are deprived of opportunity to give or to receive. However, a thread which runs consistently through Frankl's writings is that:

> *'the true meaning of life is to be found in the world rather than within man or his own psyche, as though it were a closed system.'*

Self-transcendence, the moving out and beyond the concerns of self, endow the life of the person with a deeper apprehension of meaning than self-actualisation; a notion supported by another qualified by long-term deprivation of all kinds:

> *'We cannot know ourselves or declare ourselves human unless we share in the humanity of another.' (Keenan 1992)*

Csikszentmihalyi (1992) in his discourse on optimal life experience, endorses and amplifies the above conception. He offers a simple but rich etymology of the word 'meaning', which is of such import for the occupational therapist that it might best be recounted verbatim:

> *'Its first usage points towards the end, purpose, significance of something, as in:* What is the meaning of life? *This sense of the word reflects the assumption that events are linked to each other in terms of an ultimate goal; that there is a temporal order, a causal connection between them. It assumes that phenomena are not random, but fall into recognisable*

patterns directed by a final purpose. The second usage of the word refers to a person's intentions: She usually means well. *What this sense of meaning implies is that people reveal their purposes in action; that their goals are expressed in predictable, consistent and orderly ways. Finally, the third sense in which the word is used refers to ordering information, as when one says:* Otorhinolaryngology means the study of ear, nose and throat, *or:* Red sky in the evening means good weather in the morning. *This sense of meaning points to the identity of different words, the relationship between events, and thus it helps to clarify, to establish order among related or conflicting information.'*

In sum then, we might propose that *meaning is the establishing of order and relationship in life events via the active pursuit of goals* – a definition of real utility to the occupational therapist in its emphasis on purpose in action, in doing, in acting upon the world. Indeed, Csikszentmihalyi suggests that creating meaning involves bringing order to the contents of the mind by integrating one's actions into a unified flow experience (flow being joy, creativity, the process of total involvement with life). This is potentially a helpful directive for the therapeutic relationship, implying that integrity of mind and body can be ordered through personal efforts alone, or with therapeutic assistance.

Csikszentmihalyi adds a coda to his discussion on purpose, which is to observe that purpose alone is insufficient: it must result in what he calls strivings – in an attitude of resolve – towards the goal. He believes that it is not the goal, nor even the achieving of the goal, which is important necessarily; it is the process, the 'doing', the resolution in pursuit of the goal that counts. There are echoes here of the earlier exploration of the word occupation. Seizing, laying hold of, engaging with, possessing, conquering and subduing are all pursuits deeply permeated with a sense of resolution of purpose. Csikszentmihalyi also notes that when goals are pursued with resolution, harmony and inner congruence are the result. We can pursue this idea of tension and of striving into the context of creativity.

OCCUPATION AND CREATIVITY

Rather surprisingly, the concept of creativity features very little in the occupational therapy literature. One reason for this might well be that, as with the concept of occupation itself, it is so familiar that it is taken for granted. Another reason might be that it has in a sense gone out of fashion. The little that is available in the professional literature is predominantly from the early writers, and is most frequently discussed in the context of crafts and craftsmanship – the underlying idea being that it is good for people to do or to make things with their hands. These ideas were not articulated very clearly or very convincingly, and it would appear that they fell into disrepute during the middle years of the last century, when fundamental occupational techniques were rejected as not being sufficiently scientific for the new scientific era. However, it is our personal view that in our failure to pursue a deeper understanding of creativity, we have lost a rich and powerful dynamic within occupational therapy. Creativity is not craftwork; neither should it be construed simply in terms of the things we make with our hands – the products of those manually skilled and dextrous. As May (1959) has declared:

> 'We are not dealing with hobbies, with do-it-yourself movements, holiday painting, or other forms of leisure time. ... Nowhere has the meaning of creativity been more disastrously lost than in the idea that it is something you use only on Sundays.'

Since occupational therapists have failed to give due attention to the matter of creativity, it is necessary to draw on the work of commentators from other traditions. Most are in agreement that creativity is something profoundly fundamental to the order of life; that it is, in essence, the process of bringing something new to birth, into being. Rogers (1959) has spoken for many with his contention that in any act of creativity there must be an observable product, and that the product must be of novel construction. He has thus defined the creative process as:

> '... the emergence in action of a novel relational product, growing out of the uniqueness of the individual on the one hand, and the materials, events, people or circumstances of his life on the other.'

Rogers' use of the phrase 'observable product' here is perhaps a little unhelpful, for it does elicit an image of a nicely turned pottery vase. He is, however, clear that such a 'product' might equally be the discovery of a new procedure in relationship, or the new formings of one's own personality; it need not be a tangible, concrete structure. Along with other authors, he stresses that the real essence of creativity lies in action, in doing, and not merely in novel thinking. May (1959) also addresses this idea, suggesting that it is not strictly proper to speak of a creative person, with its implication that the person has talent. A person may have talent and not use it creatively. Creativity is a process, a doing, and is known in creative action alone. Implicit in these ideas is an understanding that it is the fundamental nature of humankind to be creative; that it is not the order of genius, nor the province of the select few, but that creative activity is the essence of human life and being. Without doubt, early occupational therapists grasped this idea, acknowledging creativity as a primitive evolutionary instinct for exploration and mastery of the environment:

> 'We have only to glance back through the ages to see that necessity demanded the invention of tools and equipment required for daily living. Then, with the artistic and creative urge inherent in men, came the beautifying and decorating of these crude utensils, the development of pottery, fabrics and the resulting dignity and recognition.' (Slagle & Robeson 1941)

Even in this note, however, there is the tacit assumption that the creativity lies predominantly in the aesthetic, the 'beautifying and decorating'. There was a failure to appreciate the broader parameters of the concept.

May (1959) opens out those boundaries with his thesis on 'encounter', a concept that has much to challenge the occupational therapist.

May proposes that the creative act is first and foremost an *encounter*, a meeting – a meeting of painter and landscape, toddler and sandpit, climber and mountain, baker and yeast. The second element of the creative act is the *intensity* of the encounter. May notes that the quality of engagement in the encounter is characterised by a heightened awareness, and uses the words 'absorption', 'being caught up in', 'wholly involved' in description. He suggests that the person creating is the person intensively committed in his conscious living. These descriptors of full and wholehearted engagement, and richness of experience, are reminiscent of those applied to the word 'occupation' as alluded to earlier in this chapter; and we might pose the question as to whether occupation and creativity are perhaps two sides of the same coin, the existence of the one being a necessary condition for the existence of the other. Lastly, May suggests that 'encounter' is not simply a meeting of subject and object. He describes it as a meeting between two poles (the dynamic balance of wellness?), the objective pole of the dialectical relationship being the world. By world, he means not simply the environment, but 'the pattern of meaningful relations in which the person exists, and in the design of which he participates'. This idea resonates with Frankl's assertion that meaning can only be truly understood in the context of a person's relationship with the world (Frankl 1963):

'... *world is interrelated to the existing person at every moment. A continual dialectical process goes on between world and self, and self and world; one implies the other, and neither can be defined if we omit the other.*'

Rogers (1959) believes that these issues are of momentous import to the human species. He notes the dearth of creativity within our culture; that we educate people to conformity and stereotypy; that leisure is predominantly passive entertainment and regimented group action; that science is peopled with an abundance of technicians, but few thinkers; that industry quenches creative endeavour for the masses. He contends that the withering of a creative spirit in society constitutes an ominous threat to the survival of humankind. Other commentators concur. Torrance (1970) and Murray (1960) are both of the opinion that humanity's present troubles are largely the result of a deficiency in creative imagination, and that unless the current generation addresses this matter, future generations are at risk of extermination.

If such portentous assertions are valid, then it behoves those of us engaged in the health and welfare of persons generally – i.e. educators, therapists, psychologists, social workers, etc. – to give urgent consideration to the fostering of creativity in those for whom we have responsibility. It is our strong conviction that these assertions are valid. And we believe that for the person with dementia, wellbeing lies in the expression of his own unique creativity.

Fromm (1959) has postulated four conditions in which creativity can function. First, it requires of a person the capacity to be puzzled, to wonder, to question. Then, an ability to concentrate is needed; this is not just an attending to, but rather like May's intensity of encounter, is an attitude of full commitment. The ability to accept and deal with the conflict and tensions resulting from polarity is a third condition; and again we hear echoes of that dynamic balance of wellness:

> 'There is a general superstition that conflicts are harmful and that they should be avoided. The opposite is true. Conflicts are the source of wondering, of the development of strength, of what used to be called "character".'

Lastly, Fromm describes a condition in which one is 'willing to be born every day'. By this he suggests that being born is a process of letting go that continues outside the womb: letting go of the breast, the hand, the lap, indeed all one's certainties, to a position of reliance upon one's own creativity. Fromm considers the whole process of life as a process of birth, and that most people die before they are born: 'Creativeness means to be born before one dies'. Willingness to be born, Fromm asserts, requires courage and faith: 'Education for creativity is nothing short of education for living' (Fromm 1959).

Rogers offers three ways in which the above conditions may be set, and creatively fostered. These are that the person must be accepted as of unconditional worth; then, this acceptance must be provided in a context in which external evaluation is absent, and in which complete freedom of symbolic expression is permitted. In other words, the person is to be valued, and this is likely to occur in situations where others do not impose their own moral judgements, and where the locus of evaluation is within self. This provides for a sense of psychological safety in which the person has complete freedom to think, feel and be as she truly is.

This contention is both an affirmation and a challenge to occupational therapy. It affirms the person-centred and person-led approach that is at the heart of clinical intervention – the locus of evaluation and therefore the personal responsibility for wellness lying within the person rather than the therapist. The challenge to therapy, we believe, is in how to allow and encourage the client or patient the freedom to construct his own solutions to problems. Occupational therapists have often been prescriptive, particularly in the field of physical handicap. Therapists who have worked in this area are only too familiar with the client whose house is full of unused equipment lying in corners, gathering dust; the occupational therapist has been prescriptive (this aid will solve that problem), when in fact, when left to himself, the client usually devises his own solution to the difficulty, and it often involves a rejection of the aid. Prescriptiveness can cultivate dependence, can exacerbate disability. The therapist needs to learn to recognise and foster the innate creativity within individuals, and trust that they will, aided or unaided, bring to birth the solution that is right for them alone.

We will hold on to this view of creativity, and to these ideas of movement and striving in action as we explore the concept of wellbeing, a concept which we believe is critical to our understanding of occupational therapy in dementia care.

OCCUPATION AND WELLBEING

With its prime concern in matters of function, occupational therapy has not given priority to the matter of human wellbeing, and the nature of its relationship to occupation. We therefore need to turn again to psychology – the seminal work of Bradburn (1969) being probably the most substantial contribution on the matter. The main body of Bradburn's empirical work relates to the construction of a model of human wellbeing, which he believes exists in a balance between positive and negative affect. However, for the purposes of this discussion, what is more important is his identification of those variables which influence positive and negative affect. His findings, that positive affect is related to 'the degree to which an individual is involved in the environment around him, social contact, and active interest in the world', provide the first empirical support we have for the notion that there is some equivalence between occupation and wellbeing. And in the context of the specific variables he measured, those which had the highest correlation to positive affect were those that involved new or varied experiences. Novelty is a key concept in his assertions regarding engagement.

The work of Csikszentmihalyi and his associates on play and 'flow' (see 'Occupation and meaning', above) also focuses on this concept of novelty in experience. To be sure, his prime concern is optimal experience, but if we make the reasonable assumption that optimal experience is the apotheosis of wellbeing, then the work is very relevant to this discussion. Csikszentmihalyi's model of optimal experience (1975) is built around the notion of a balance between challenges and skills. A radical simplification of the model suggests that:

- low skills and low challenges are the setting for apathy
- low skills and high challenges result in anxiety
- high skills and low challenges lead to boredom
- high skills and high challenges are the route to optimal experience.

A later refining of this model (Massimini & Carli 1988) suggests that for optimal experience to occur, skills and challenges do not merely need to be in balance, they need to be in balance *above* the level which is customary for the individual. In other words, the pianist will not know optimal experience while playing a piece at which he is competent, such will only occur when he is mastering that difficult piece which is stretching him beyond his previous limits – in effect, when he is engaging with a new experience which requires a new skill. It seems reasonable to suggest then, on the basis of the extensive empirical work underpinning both the above models, that wellbeing cannot be understood except in the context of an active engagement with the world, and that degree of wellbeing is determined by the extent to which that engagement is in the context of novel and varied experience.

Much has been made in this chapter of the notion of a seizing for oneself, a striving in action, as having some equivalence to wellness and wellbeing, and there are probably few who would not concur with this as an underpinning tenet of occupational therapy generally. But a question we must ask here is whether such a concept is helpful or relevant to the person who has dementia, whose skills and abilities are radically circumscribed, and on the decline. Can we truly expect a person whose cognitive function is distorted and dysfunctional, to pursue and engage, to seize and to strive, to encounter and 'give birth'? Yes, we can. But in order to do so, we must come away from the traditional rehabilitative concepts noted earlier, viz. self-actualisation, autonomy, independence. These terms become increasingly redundant in the context of an advancing dementia.

We are dealing here with a degenerative condition. People are not going to get better; generally speaking, we expect them to get worse. As far as our current body of knowledge informs us, we understand that dementia is not an illness from which one may recover through a facilitation of natural healing processes. It is perhaps more accurate to think in terms of analogy with an autoimmune condition; the programme is set at self-destruct, only in this case it is the psyche which is at stake, not the body. There is a sense then, in which we are working against the flow of a natural order, rather than with it.

Traditionally, occupational therapy is carried out with the minimum possible intervention from the therapist, and always with the aim of ultimate withdrawal to ensure the independence and self-sufficiency of the client. This is where, in dementia care, we must depart from convention. For effective occupational intervention in dementia care can only be understood in the context of the interface between therapist and client; wellbeing in dementia care can only be understood in the context of the interface between therapist and client. *This is the key.* And this is what we shall be at pains to stress throughout this book.

In order to establish and develop a therapeutic process in the context of dementia, two things are necessary. First and foremost, we must understand the changing world of the dementing person; there is a very real sense in which the dementing person inhabits a different world to the one you and I live in, and we need to get under the skin of this. Then, we must have a clear appreciation of the critical partnership between carer and dementing person which is at the seat of wellbeing in dementia. Chapter 3 attempts to explore the world of the person who has dementia, and Chapter 4 examines the significance of the carer role to health and wellbeing.

Key Points

- Occupational therapists have struggled to practise effectively in dementia care.
- This struggle is due to inadequacies in our use and development of occupational theory in relation to the problems we need to tackle.
- Traditional models of adaptation and rehabilitation are not helpful.
- A broader understanding of occupation as 'that which we possess and which possesses us', provides a more fitting basis for developing a workable paradigm.

- A state of 'wellness' rather than of 'health' is a more appropriate goal in dementia care, because it is found in dynamic process rather than in fixed state.
- Creativity is profoundly fundamental to the order of life, and modern-day occupational therapists have lost a rich and powerful therapeutic dynamic in failing to acknowledge its critical place in occupational theory.
- Wellbeing is nurtured in creative expression, though psychological safety is a necessary condition for creativity to function.
- There is clear empirical support for the notion of an equivalence between occupation and wellbeing.
- Optimum wellbeing exists in a balance of skills and challenges above an individual's customary level.
- The convention within occupational therapy of minimal intervention and withdrawal from the client is not tenable in dementia care.
- A therapeutic process in the context of dementia requires an understanding of the changing world of the dementing person, as well as an appreciation of the relationship between that person and their carer(s).

References

Berry C, Berry M 1984 Wellness: a positive strategy for a healthy business. Time Magazine, Special Advertising Section, June 18th

Bradburn N 1969 The structure of psychological well-being. Aldine, Chicago

Capra F 1982 The turning point: science, society and the rising culture. Simon and Schuster, New York

Cousins N 1979 Anatomy of an illness as perceived by the patient. W W Norton, New York

Csikszentmihalyi M 1975 Beyond boredom and anxiety. Jossey-Bass, San Francisco

Csikszentmihalyi M 1992 Flow: the psychology of happiness. Rider, London

Dubos R 1980 Man adapting. Yale University Press, New Haven, CT

Engelhardt H 1983 Occupational therapists as technologists and custodians of meaning. In: Kielhofner G (ed) Health through occupation. F A Davis, Philadelphia

Frankl V 1963 Man's search for meaning. Washington Square, New York

Fromm E 1959 The creative attitude. In: Anderson H (ed) Creativity and its cultivation. Harper & Row, New York

Gordon I 1958 That damned word health. Lancet ii: 638–639

Hagedorn R 1995 Occupational therapy: perspectives and processes. Churchill Livingstone, Edinburgh

Illich I 1975 Medical nemesis: the expropriation of health. Calder & Boyars, London

Johnson J 1986 Wellness: a context for living. Slack, NJ

Keenan B 1992 An evil cradling. London, Vintage

Massimini F, Carli M 1988 The systematic assessment of flow in daily experience. In: Csikszentmihalyi M, Csikszentmihalyi I (eds) Optimal experience. Cambridge University Press, Cambridge

May R 1959 The nature of creativity. In: Anderson H (ed) Creativity and its cultivation. Harper & Row, New York

Morton I, Bleathman C 1988 Does it matter whether it's Tuesday or Friday? Nursing Times 84(6):25–27

Murray H 1960 A mythology for grown-ups. Saturday Review 43(4):10–12

Naisbitt J 1982 Megatrends: ten new directions transforming our lives. Warner Books, New York

Opatz J 1985 A primer of health promotion. Oryn Publications, Washington, DC

Reilly M 1962 Occupational therapy can be one of the great ideas of 20th century medicine. American Journal of Occupational Therapy XVI (1):1–9

Rogers C 1959 Towards a theory of creativity. In: Anderson H (ed) Creativity and its cultivation. Harper & Row, New York

Sharrott G 1983 Occupational therapy's role in the client's creation and affirmation of meaning. In: Kielhofner G (ed) Health through occupation. F A Davis, Philadelphia

Slagle E, Robeson H 1941 Syllabus for training of nurses in occupational therapy. State Hospitals Press, New York

Torrance E 1970 Causes for concern. In: Vernon P (ed) Creativity: selected readings. Penguin, Harmondsworth

Chapter 3

The altered world of dementia

It is of course impossible for most of us to enter in any significant way into the world of the person who has cognitive impairments. Probably only those who have suffered a temporary memory loss or a transient confusional state, or some other altered state of consciousness, can even begin to understand what it must be like. But this is something that as carers of people with dementia we must try to do, for it is only as we have some measure of appreciation of the subjective experience that we can begin to respond appropriately.

We know that the person with dementia is unlikely to remember things in the way that they used to, or to be able to concentrate well; that language and comprehension may become muddled, and so on. This is the outward evidence of that with which we are all too familiar; but is there any way of exploring how the world is changing for that person, how it might be viewed from their point of view? We think that there is. There is of course much scope for improving our understanding, but we have found a fairly simple analogy to be a helpful starting point.

There has been considerable support over the years for the notion that the cognitive losses of dementia reflect (in a reverse direction) the cognitive gains of childhood; and a name that crops up repeatedly in the literature is that of the Swiss psychologist Piaget. Numerous commentators have found in Piaget's intricate theory of cognitive development, a mirroring of dementia's cognitive decline.

From the psychology literature, the work of de Ajuriaguerra et al (1964), using Piagetian tests on elderly people who have dementia, was the first to make such a link: 'we have found in our patients all the stages of childhood described by Piaget'. More recently, Reisberg's (1986) diagnostic 'staging' tool for Alzheimer's disease (FAST) supports their hypothesis that deficits in dementia represent a reversal of Piaget's developmental stages. The experiments of Stuart-Hamilton & McDonald (1996) using Piagetian tasks with unimpaired subjects, strengthen such a hypothesis. Most of this literature has been concerned with functional assessment alone, and indeed, a number of attempts have been made to construct assessment instruments based on a Piagetian hierarchy (McCurren & Ganong 1984, Cole & Dastoor 1987, Sclan et al 1990).

Piaget has also influenced the occupational therapy literature, though in considerably smaller measure. Würsten (1974) suggested that a Piagetian model of development had much to offer the concept of adaptation in occupational therapy. Unfortunately, he omitted to say how. Landsmann & Katz (1988) attempted to apply a Piagetian framework of assessment tests to psychiatric patients, but failed to offer a rationale for their assumption that developmental regression is at the root of mental illness. Both of these theories appear to have disappeared without trace in subsequent literature.

A much weightier contribution to professional advancement has been Mosey's (1986) developmental frame of reference for occupational therapy, which is underpinned in some measure by Piagetian theory in its sequential linking of skills to stages of chronological development. Rather like Reisberg's FAST instrument, it is designed to 'stage' an individual at a certain level of development and functional ability. Unlike the FAST, it is neither age- nor condition-specific, and is proposed for the field of mental health generally, to act as an indicator of functional level and as a guide for the appropriate delivery of therapy.

Also using Piaget as a base theory is the cognitive disability model of Allen (1985), whose six levels of cognitive ability are influenced by Piagetian concepts. This model was designed for occupational therapy with all cognitive disabilities, and this necessarily includes dementia, though Conroy's (1996) evaluation of the model found the cognitive levels poorly articulated, and the model as a whole of limited utility in severe dementia.

A common thread running throughout this selection of literature is its primary concern with function and the assessment of function; it all appears to be driven by the question, 'At what level of function is this impaired person now operating?'. We can make use of this material for assessment purposes if we wish, but we feel that it is actually more useful as an exploratory tool. That is how we shall use it in this chapter.

What appears to have been largely neglected in the body of literature surrounding Piaget's work, is a study of the activity context in which his children developed their functional abilities, and the notion that such activity might actually be used in the context of therapeutic practice. A question which appears not to have been asked is, 'If a person is at a given level of functioning, how might therapy be organised to accommodate that person?'. Chapter 8 looks specifically at this question.

Piaget was a prolific writer, with a very complex style, and in order to distil the key features of his theory, we have attempted a summary of his principal contentions. He categorised cognitive development in the child into four main stages (reflex, sensorimotor, representational, reflective), covering the ages 0–15. Each stage is again subdivided to demonstrate the progressive acquisition of cognitive skills as far as the individual's mid-teens, at which point development is conceived to be complete. The following list is presented in reverse order to that set out by Piaget, i.e. 15 years (development complete) to 0 years (undeveloped), in order to offer a picture of cognitive decline as it might be viewed in dementia.

Formal Operational (11–15 years) – maturity of thought

- Operations initiated in cooperation with others.
- Hypothetico-deductive reasoning – a problem is considered in terms of all possible relations that could hold true. All hypotheses are confirmed or rejected via experimentation.
- Propositional thinking – the ability to manipulate raw data into organised statements/propositions.
- Interpropositional thinking – the ability to develop logical relationships between propositions.
- Simplifying rules are devised to facilitate solutions to problems.
- Reflective thought is developed, and thought relating to future events is well articulated.

Concrete Operational (7–11 years) – mastery of classes, relations, numbers

- Operations characterised by a decrease in egocentricity from former stages, and an increase in cooperation.
- Mobility of thinking:
  - ability to deploy reversibility (to consider a series of reverse operations that will restore an original situation)
  - ability to decentre (to appreciate more than one stimulus at a time)
  - ability to take another's role
  - ability to conceptualise class relations.
- Ability to utilise relational terms – e.g. bigger/darker.
- Seriation – ability to arrange objects in terms of weight, size, etc.
- Mental representation of seriation (ability to take overall view of whole series of actions taken to complete a task, e.g. a mental picture of each stage of the route to school).

Preoperational – Intuitive (4–7 years) – mastery of symbol

- Rudimentary concept of class (based on perceptual similarity, not logic, e.g. a starfish might be classed as a rock).
- Irreversibility of thought – see above.
- Inability to acknowledge conservation (that quantities of liquid/mass remain invariant in the face of perceptual transformation – e.g. a pint of water in a long tall glass is perceived to be greater in volume than a pint in a short fat glass).
- Lack of direction in thinking (unrelated explanations of the causes of an event juxtaposed).
- Egocentric thinking – human qualities attributed to natural phenomena.
- Difficulty in understanding simple relations, particularly in regard to self – e.g. bigger/smaller, left/right.

Preoperational – Preconceptual (2–4 years) – genesis of conceptual thought

- Linguistic development and ability to construct symbols (enabling past experience to be applied to present events).
- Syncretism (tendency to group unrelated events or items into a whole – e.g. woman, cookies, clock, matches = kitchen).

■ Egocentric thought (thinking only from own point of view – no ability to take the role of another).

■ Centring (ability to focus on only one aspect of a stimulus array at a time – others overlooked).

■ World events perceived to have been caused by people (e.g. daylight caused by switching the light on).

Sensorimotor (0–2 years) – mastery of concrete objects

■ Internal experimentation (18 months to 2 years). Utilisation of mental symbols to refer to objects absent from the immediate environment. Solutions to problems considered in a mental dimension rather than a physical (e.g. object will be sought where it last disappeared from view, rather than where it was last hidden).

■ Tertiary circular reactions (1 year to 18 months). Object permanence established. Exploration of objects/events by trial and error experimentation. Interest in novel variation and how that variation affects objects or ability to obtain objects (e.g. toy under a pillow will be obtained by indirect measures such as kicking the pillow or displacing it with a stick).

■ Secondary reactions (8 to 12 months). Means/ends clearly differentiated. Simple problem-solving. Beginnings of object permanence (a toy under a pillow continues to exist and will be sought; it is not 'out-of-sight-out-of-mind' as in the earlier stage).

■ Secondary circular reactions (4 to 8 months). Manipulation of events/objects in the external environment; repetitive as in earlier stage, but now because of the interesting stimulus effects of the activity (e.g. arm-waving to move a toy suspended over a pram).

■ Primary circular reactions (0 to 4 months). Non-intentional spontaneous actions centring on the body (thumb-sucking/blanket plucking), repeated for their own sake.

■ Reflex (0 to 1 month). Externally evoked or self-initiated (sucking, grasping). Sympathetic crying.

Before proceeding, it should perhaps be noted that in the years since Piaget published his findings, there has been an extensive and vigorous debate on their validity as a model of cognitive development. His 'stage' structure has come under particular criticism (Flavell 1963, Cohen 1983), as have most of the experimental scenarios with his children upon which he formulated his conclusions (Donaldson 1978, Cohen 1983).

Data emerging from subsequent research suggest that Piaget significantly underestimated the abilities of young children, and often overestimated the abilities of teenagers. The principal criticism is not so much that growing children do not pass through developmental hierarchies of object permanence, egocentricity, conservation, class relationship, etc., but that they pass through them rather differently, and at different levels of experience to those which Piaget suggests. One of Piaget's main contentions was that children learn predominantly through the manipulation of their bodies and objects in the environment. Thought, logical thought, was the pre-eminent product, and was the determining factor in emotional and social experience (Cowan 1978). A child could only feel those feelings and engage in those relationships that his cognitive skills determined. Subsequent research suggests otherwise:

- The work of Zajonc et al (1989) suggests that cognitive appraisal need not necessarily feature at all in emotion at its most elemental level.
- Bryant & Trabasso (1972) demonstrated logical ability in children at a much earlier stage than Piaget allowed.
- Harris (1975) found that children could handle concepts earlier than Piaget ruled.
- Maratsos (1976), Lloyd (1975) and Hughes (1975) conducted experiments which demonstrated that young children are, under certain circumstances, able to appreciate the point of view of another, and not as egocentric as Piaget would suggest.
- The work of Wolff (1963) and Carpenter (1974) also challenged this contention, finding evidence of appreciation of the human face even in very young babies. Rosenthal (1982) suggested that some social interaction is evident at 3 days.

There are many other studies. Indeed, the 1970s seems to be a decade dedicated to the rejection of as many of Piaget's claims as possible. What is particularly interesting, however, is that none of these studies invalidates Piaget's theory, nor refutes his claims out of hand. What they do achieve, in pointing up his omissions, is a highlighting of matters of critical importance to those concerned with child development. For example, information must make sense to a child, and be culturally appropriate, for him to be able to mobilise appropriately those skills at his disposal. The way a situation is described and materials presented, has a considerable impact upon a child's comprehension of a task. Thus, social setting (the people involved in a situation) also has a bearing on the ability to accomplish tasks. Training is important; a child's familiarity with materials and procedures will maximise the demonstration of his abilities.

Clearly, optimum environmental circumstances are critical for the child's acquisition and demonstration of cognitive skills. This was Piaget's greatest omission. His research took place in the context of what was, by all accounts, a stable family relationship (his own), and he failed to appreciate fully the influence that secure, underpinning relationships have on satisfactory development. Attachment theory (see Ch. 4) has made good this deficit, and supports the assertion of Goldfarb (1943, 1947) and Winnicott (1971) that a reliable, constant caregiver is a critical feature of early childhood development.

Practitioners in dementia care need to heed this material. Not only does it supplement our discussion of how elderly people may operate, particularly in the latter stages of a dementia, it also offers a sense of hope, in that if we can optimise environmental circumstances and cues in the way that child care has for the child, we might be able to facilitate communication in a far more significant way in those whose cognitive abilities are greatly diminished. Piaget's model offers us a base theory. Perhaps we in dementia care, like those in child psychology before us, need not only to examine the theory and its application, but also to undertake a broad research interest in the surrounding 'microenvironment' as it impacts upon people who are severely impaired.

Although Piaget structured his theory in developmental phases, and believed that a person could not move on to stage three before stage two had been achieved, he was nevertheless concerned not to imply that individuals suddenly switched from one step to another in a stepwise fashion, and he promoted the notion of a steadily cumulative acquisition of cognitions – skill upon skill. It is this pattern, we believe, which has much to offer our perception of the dementing process.

Those who care for people with dementia over the long term are only too familiar with a picture of slow progressive decline. This is perhaps particularly the case for those relatives who care for a loved one at home for an extended period. It is they who pick up the first perhaps trivial inconsistencies; they who must accommodate and adapt as those inconsistencies magnify and multiply. Clearly, impairments do not arrive in stages, but without doubt in many people there is a familiar cumulative pattern of loss over time. We would contend that Piaget's model of cognitive gain, viewed in reverse, is a helpful guide for understanding the cognitive losses of dementia as a slowly progressive bereavement of acquired skill and ability. Such a proposition is not intended to imply a *regression* to childhood or childishness, for there are many unknowns in dementia, and where the child has no experience, no history, the elderly person has vast amounts of both, and we will never be quite sure how much of that is cognitively retained. Bereavement is a better word. When we lose a loved relative or friend, *we* have not regressed, we simply no longer have them with us in actuality. We have memory, visual image, and possibly pain and grief because of those images. But our essential selves have not changed; it is simply that our human condition is impoverished, we are poorer people for the loss of a rich resource in our life. We believe that it is so with the cognitive bereavement of dementia.

So what are the results of this impoverishment for the person concerned? How is the world changing for them? It might be helpful to explore Piaget's categories of development with reference to the last few years of Brian Wallace, who died recently at the age of 71.

Brian was 63 years of age when things started to go wrong. He had been the headmaster of the local primary school for the last 15 years, and was a very able man, quick-thinking and decisive. He had a democratic style of management, and important decisions concerning the school were always opened up to the staff team. Staff knew that their opinions would always be considered, although one or two of the more senior staff privately felt that Brian had often made up his mind on a matter even before calling a staff meeting. He was very adept at setting out all the angles of a problem, and drawing out of his colleagues a range of possible solutions, but he was a good manipulator too, and could invariably argue his own case to a satisfactory conclusion.

It was actually Brian's school colleagues (not his wife, Louise, as might have been expected) who were the first to notice changes, and it was the staff meetings where the problems first showed up. For the first time in his life it seemed to Brian as though his brain hadn't got its usual capacity;

he couldn't hold on to the volume of information under discussion, and he knew from comments that were made that he was forgetting things, or rather, that things were just bypassing him, and not sinking in, in the first place. He was finding it difficult to follow the thread of an argument; his thinking seemed slow and sluggish and he couldn't keep up. The cut and thrust of debate which he would once have enjoyed being in the thick of now frightened and embarrassed him. He gradually contributed less and less, and delegated more of the team leadership and decision making to his senior staff.

He found too that his secretary was getting very irritable with him these days. She was forever reminding him of times of appointments and meetings, as though he had suddenly become incompetent. Several times he had even found appointments in the diary that he had not asked her to make. She was taking too much into her own hands; he would have to speak to her about it. And when Councillor Watts had turned up out of the blue for what he said was a three-way meeting with himself and the deputy head, he began to wonder if there was some conspiracy afoot.

It wasn't until three staff in the same day had asked him if he felt unwell, that Brian sat down and took stock. No, he wasn't himself, he knew that. Something was going wrong inside his head. It was school that was the problem. He was fine at home, nothing had changed there; it was the pace of life at school that was getting to him. He saw the doctor, who talked a lot about stress and anxiety and overdoing it, and recommended that he took time off sick. He thought a complete break and a holiday was probably what he needed.

The holiday didn't go well. He and Louise had arranged to return to their usual hotel in the Greek islands, but when they arrived it was the wrong one. Louise was adamant that it wasn't, that this was the hotel they always stayed in, but Brian didn't remember any of it. He got very angry with the courier, and wondered if there was some plot between him and Louise. He eventually agreed to stay for one night because it was so late anyway; as Louise pointed out, it was an extremely nice hotel, and it wasn't going to cost them any more than what they had already paid. Louise talked to him the following morning about what she called his memory problem. It made him feel very uncomfortable, but he had to admit that he wasn't himself, and he realised that he was upsetting Louise. But he was upset too; nothing was familiar and he felt lost; he longed to be at home. They returned a week early.

Brian was not able to return to work, and ultimately took early retirement. Louise hung on to her part-time job for a while and tried to encourage Brian to take on some of the household tasks. He was always happy to go shopping, and increasingly this was becoming the major event of the day. The supermarket was only four streets away, but Brian found that he didn't have a picture of the route in his head. Some days he would set off and suddenly realise that he didn't recognise anything; he'd keep going, too embarrassed to turn back and admit it to Louise, and more often than not he would come across it sooner or later. Occasionally he would recognise a familiar feature such as the church, and the rusty old car without wheels, but he had no concept of the area as a whole.

Sometimes he realised that he wasn't even doing the shopping very well. Louise would complain that he brought back things she hadn't asked for, and she often said she never could understand where all the money went. They had started to have rows about this, and eventually, it was just easier not to do it at all.

After the episode of the flooded bathroom, Louise gave up her job. Thrown increasingly upon each other's company, relationships became strained. Louise became irritable; Brian couldn't seem to remember what she had just told him, and would repeat the same question over and over. He could say what he wanted for dinner, or what he wanted to see on TV, but was no longer able to discuss the state of the world as they once used to, nor express an opinion on the news events of the day. Louise missed their discussions.

Brian had stopped attending the local writers' club when someone had laughed at his latest piece of writing. Reading it, Louise found that it was indeed garbled and nonsensical. She tried to encourage him to continue his writing at home, but he seemed no longer to have any ideas, and had little concentration. He would get angry at her urging, and eventually Louise gave up, feeling that the anger probably arose from a partial insight that he could no longer do what he once did well. She was aware that he couldn't use language verbally as he once did either. He often struggled to find words to express himself; nouns seemed to be a particular problem and there was a growing vagueness and repetitiveness about the words and phrases he used.

The gardening they continued to do together, and it gave Brian pleasure. Louise had found that he was more comfortable these days with simple practical tasks; tasks that required him to use his body and didn't require much thought. It didn't matter if the occasional prize bloom was pulled up and consigned to the compost heap. He could no longer remember the names of the flowers and plants, or how to use trowel and hoe properly, but would often recount a 'Flower Show' reminiscence again and again. Louise would try to remember to laugh at the punch line on each occasion. Latterly Brian would just sit and watch as Louise did the gardening; she preferred it that way, it was easier.

Some of Brian's friends were no longer in touch. Louise put it down to embarrassment. Bob and Vera still came though, and were very supportive. Brian rarely recognised them now and usually greeted them, if at all, as new acquaintances. They never stayed long; Brian wasn't able to join the conversation; sometimes he didn't seem to know they were there, sometimes he became agitated and abusive. But the visits helped Louise.

Louise no longer took Brian out with her. She didn't drive, and his agitation and shouting on the bus on the last two occasions they had gone into town, had embarrassed and upset her badly. So she mostly stayed home, where Brian now followed her every move, from room to room, even to the toilet. It seemed that if she wasn't directly in view, he would believe himself abandoned. The only respite she got was when the carer from the sitting service came and sat with him, and she would have a few hours to herself. The look of relief on Brian's face and the occasional tears on her return, made her feel guilty. Louise began to feel that a very real role change was taking place; these days their relationship seemed more like mother and son than husband and wife. She felt disloyal for thinking this way, but that's how it was.

During the winter of Brian's 68th birthday, Louise's health broke. She spent 2 weeks in hospital, and a further month with Bob and Vera convalescing. Brian was taken into The Elms residential home the day after Louise was admitted to hospital, and it was 4 weeks before she saw him again. Bob drove her over shortly after she returned from hospital. They found him in a chair in the corner of the room; he didn't recognise either of them. When she was able to return home, Louise started visiting every day. This seemed to make a difference; sometimes Brian would recognise her and return her affection, but sometimes he wouldn't. He could no longer put coherent sentences together, and he would converse in a sort of gobbledegook that she couldn't understand, but would try and enter into. Occasionally he would give a one-word or one-phrase response appropriately to a question. 'How are you today?' 'Fed up!' 'How was the outing yesterday?' 'Alright.'

Such occasions grew increasingly rare. From time to time when she visited, she would find that Brian had been included in a group that was playing ball with a member of staff. Initially she felt humiliated for him; this was very demeaning and she took it up with the staff. They asked her just to sit and watch next time a group took place, which she did. And she noticed that Brian was indeed different on these occasions. There seemed to be something pleasurable for him in repeated movements over and over again. In fact she was reminded of last year's Christmas party, when he got such a childlike pleasure from those balloons. And there was no question that he was smiling a lot as well, and moving about in his chair, neither of which she was able to get him to do on the occasions of her usual visits.

Eventually Brian stopped speaking altogether, only making occasional noises. Louise would visit every lunchtime and help him with his dinner. It helped the staff a little, and it helped her to have something concrete to do. She could talk to him, hold his hand and stroke his hair, but most of the time his eyes were glazed and unseeing, and Louise felt that she might as well not be there. On rare occasions his eyes would meet hers and hold her gaze, and at these times Louise felt that he knew her, that there was a thread of communication between them, and was glad she had come. She was reminded of a similar gaze of studied intensity on the face of her baby son as she held him in her arms some 40 years ago. No words were necessary then; indeed there were none. It seemed to be a gaze of communion, of oneness quite elemental in nature. Louise wondered if the end of the journey was in some way the same as the beginning, and was strangely comforted. Brian died just 3 days short of his 71st birthday.

What then are we saying about the world that Brian was living in? Well, it was a world out of control, where Brian no longer held the reins; it was a world of growing isolation, for there was no-one available to walk the road with him; it was a world of diminishing competence, as skills were slowly eroded across all areas of daily living; it was a world of distorted perception, where people and things no longer behaved in the way they used to; it was a world of increasing dependence and helplessness. Above all it was a world of chaotic emotions: bewilderment, fear, embarrassment, shame, frustration, anger, insecurity, paranoia, loneliness. Perhaps the only way we can even begin to enter in to the experience is to think back to our childhood, or to a time in adulthood when we were sick or disabled; a time when for whatever reason we were out of control, helpless, dependent and isolated. Perhaps we need to think of that occasion when we were made to feel foolish, when everybody else seemed to know what to do except us; a time when friends ganged up against us and we were 'sent to Coventry'; when we couldn't do that thing which for everybody else was so easy; when we got lost on the way home. These things are the stuff of dementia; they are, in a way, analogues of the dementing experience. It would serve us well to revisit them, and remember.

We have wondered if the journey of a dementia is not in a very real sense an analogue of a return to childhood. But this is not a popular proposition. Who amongst us can feel positive about relinquishing the benefits of adulthood in order to adopt the constraints of childhood? To be a child is to be vulnerable, to be physically weak, to have limited skills, to be under authority. To be an adult is to have control, authority, choice, to be strong, to have many skills. What adult would willingly embrace a concept of such vulnerability again? It is something to be feared. In addition, carers of people who have dementia have over recent years fought long and hard to eradicate that style of care practice which has been called 'nursery care', that style of care which patronises, demeans and infantilises. No carer worth his salt is going to allow a return to the old culture.

The concerns and anxieties around such a proposition are understandable. But it is our belief that failure to dig a little deeper into this concept is to miss a rich vein of ideas in our search for understanding. To recognise that a person has returned to a childlike level of functioning is not a licence to treat them as we might a child, in an authoritative, controlling fashion. Why should it be? Rather, it should open up new possibilities, new avenues of approach, closed to us if all we have to rely on are our adult-to-adult social mechanisms.

We have wondered if the journey of dementia might be perceived as one in which the traveller moves from a life of doing to a life of being. As the child first is, and later does, so the person with dementia first does, and then is. Michael Ignatieff (1992), from his family experience of three generations of Alzheimer's disease, has used the term 'primary self' to describe a person in the latter stages of a dementia; this is a helpful concept and one which fits well with our propositions. In an attempt to answer the question of whether the person with dementia actually becomes another, a different person, as their condition deteriorates, he says this:

> 'Carers often conclude, quite rightly, that the person they are caring for is no longer the person they once knew. But if they aren't, who have they become?
>
> Vegetables is one answer. But that's not what I see when I'm on the Alzheimer's ward of a nursing home. Vegetables are all the same. Each Alzheimer patient is very different, and all, in my experience, preserve

tiny elements of personality right to the end. I know an old woman, who can't feed herself or speak, but who continues to stare out at the world through her bifocals with the same shrewd and deeply intelligent expression of her younger years.

In the people I have known who have succumbed to the disease, there still remains, at the end, a primary and incorrigible core of selfhood. That essential self remains in their expression, their gait, some tiny habit, some gesture, some faint glint of humour, even a liking for ice cream.

They are not vegetables, but primary selves. They are no longer like us, busy and full of purposes, bent on becoming something. Instead, they are prisoners of the realm of pure being. In this realm there is only now, this instant. There is only the way the ice cream tastes when you have it on your tongue. The quiet in a nursing home is not, I think, the silence of the grave, but the peace of pure being.'

Understanding that a person is experiencing a rather different world to the one we inhabit, and that they are perceiving it in many respects with the faculties of a child, is first a challenge to reconsider our approach, our style of contact, our manner of communication. For we approach a 12-month-old rather differently to how we approach a 7-year-old. And we approach a 15-year-old differently again. Our expectations and our demands vary according to our understanding of their abilities and their perception of the world. Openness, consideration and courtesy can naturally be a constant in our approach to all age groups, but unless our expectations are modified by our appreciation of level of ability in cognitive and social skills, our interactions are likely to be unproductive. We have different expectations and use a different approach in each case.

Not only is this proposition a challenge to us to reconsider our approach, it is a challenge to rethink what being a child is all about. Being a child is about being vulnerable, to be sure, about dependence, about limited skills. But it is about so many other things too, and if all we can see is the negative, we are missing something important. Paradoxically, being a child is also about freedom: freedom from responsibility, freedom of expression, freedom to be oneself as one really is, a lack of self-consciousness and all the constraints that go with it. It is about creativity and imagination and fantasy and laughter and fun. It is about a world which most of us have long forgotten, brought up as we have been to prize above all things the cerebral over the emotional, the scientific over the artistic, the rational over the intuitive. Have we forgotten the good things about being a child? Then we need to think again. The dementing person has been bereaved of much, certainly, but it is not all loss; there are some things regained, and our task as therapists is to recognise that and to use it creatively.

Chapter 4 explores further this concept of a return to childhood, in the context of our approach as carers and therapists. How important are we in the world of the dementing person? What is our role? How should we conduct ourselves? What expectations should the dementing person have of us?

> ## Key Points
>
> - Understanding that a person is experiencing a rather different world to the one we inhabit, and that they are perceiving it in many respects as with the faculties of a child, is a challenge to reconsider our approach, our style of contact, our manner of communication.
> - There is considerable support for the proposition that the cognitive losses of the person with dementia might be understood as a reversal of early childhood cognitive stages of development.
> - Occupational therapists Mosey and Allen have both adapted developmental models for the profession, although not specifically for the field of dementia care.
> - The respective contributions of Mosey and Allen have been influenced by Piagetian theory, which categorises cognitive development into four main stages across ages 0 years (undeveloped) to 15 years (fully developed).
> - Critics of Piaget, although not rejecting his central tenet of the notion of cumulative acquisition of skill, highlight matters of critical importance such as environmental circumstances, which he failed to address.
> - In dementia care, the occupational therapist can draw from Piaget and his critics to develop: effective therapeutic intervention; knowledge about the nature of cognitive skills which may be lost; knowledge about what constitutes optimal environmental circumstances for the person who has dementia; knowledge about the critical qualities of the reliable constant caregiver so crucial to the child, and likewise therefore for the person who has dementia.

References

Allen C 1985 Occupational therapy for psychiatric diseases: measurement and management of cognitive disabilities. Little, Brown, Boston

Bryant P, Trabasso T 1972 Transitive inferences and memory in young children. Nature 232:456–458

Carpenter G 1974 Mother's face and the newborn. In: Lewis R (ed) Child alive. Temple Smith, London

Cohen D 1983 Piaget: critique and re-assessment. St Martin's Press, New York

Cole M, Dastoor D 1987 A new hierarchic approach to the measurement of dementia. Psychosomatics 28(6):298–304

Conroy C 1996 Dementia care: keeping intact and in touch. Avebury, Aldershot

Cowan P 1978 Piaget with feeling. Holt, Rinehart and Winston, New York

de Ajuriaguerra J, Bellet-Muller M, Tissot R 1964 A propos de quelques problèmes posés par le déficit opératoire de veillards atteint de démence dégénérative en début d'évolution. Cortex 1:232–256

Donaldson M 1978 Children's minds. Croom Helm, London

Flavell J 1963 The developmental psychology of Jean Piaget. Van Nostrand, London

Goldfarb W 1943 The effects of early institutional care on adolescent personality. Journal of Experimental Education 12:107–129

Goldfarb W 1947 Variations in adolescent adjustment in institutionally reared children. Journal of Orthopsychiatry 17:449–457

Harris P 1975 Inferences and semantic development. Journal of Child Language 2:143–152

Hughes M 1975 Egocentrisms in pre-school children. Unpublished PhD dissertation, University of Edinburgh

Ignatieff M 1992 A taste of ice cream is all you know. The Observer, 4th July

Landsmann L, Katz N 1988 Concrete to formal thinking: comparison of psychiatric outpatients and a normal control group. Occupational Therapy in Mental Health 1(8):73–94

Lloyd P 1975 Communication in pre-school children. Unpublished PhD dissertation, University of Edinburgh

McCurren C, Ganong L 1984 Assessing cognitive functioning of the elderly with the 'Inventory of Piaget's Developmental Tasks'. Journal of Advanced Nursing 9:449–456

Maratsos M 1976 The use of the definite and indefinite reference in young children. Cambridge University Press, Cambridge

Mosey A 1986 Psychosocial components of occupational therapy. Raven Press, New York

Reisberg B 1986 Dementia: a systematic approach to identifying reversible causes. Geriatrics 41(4):30–46

Rosenthal R 1982 Early human experience. Developmental Psychology 18:36

Sclan S, Foster J, Reisberg B, Franssen E, Welkowitz J 1990 Application of Piagetian measures of cognition in severe Alzheimer's disease. Psychiatric Journal of the University of Ottawa 15(4):221–226

Stuart-Hamilton I, McDonald L 1996 Age and a possible regression to childhood thinking patterns. PSIGE Newsletter 58:13–15

Winnicott D 1971 Playing and reality. Tavistock, London

Wolff P 1963 Observations on the early development of smiling. In: Foss B (ed) Determinants of infant behaviour 2. Methuen, London

Würsten H 1974 On the relevancy of Piaget's theory to occupational therapy. American Journal of Occupational Therapy 28(4):213–217

Zajonc R, Murphy S, Inglehart M 1989 Feeling and facial efference: implications of the vascular theory of emotion. Psychological Review 96(3):395–416

Chapter **4**

The significance of the carer

The scenario recorded in Box 4.1 was actually an informal note, scribbled 'stream of consciousness' style in the period after lunch one day. I had not long arrived on the unit, and it was written perhaps in part as abreaction. I thought that all my years in dementia care had inured me to disturbing sights and sounds; but this rattled me badly, and I felt a need to get it down on paper so that I could take it away and look at it more objectively some time when I could feel less emotional about it.

This was undeniably a bad day on the unit, and not typical of the usual order of things. Staff had been invisible for some considerable time, perhaps because this time of day in residential care, after lunch, is usually the quiet and uneventful hour when most people are having a snooze. But not today. It was a salutary experience to see what arises without the modifying presence of carers. Even more disturbing than the noise, though, was the complete and utter self-containment of each person in that room. It was as though, for each person, nobody else existed. Even Jim's contact with Hester was more in the manner of swatting a fly than a true personal interaction. It is possible that there was some communication through noise, one noise sparking off another in a reflex manner, rather as one baby crying might trigger another; but this is conjecture. Certainly there was almost no visual communication; two or three were looking around, but what they were actually perceiving or visually engaging with is a matter of question. It was only when staff returned to the unit, and started to attend to this resident and to that, that the noise very gradually started to abate, and the chaos began to come under control. Eventually, a sense of some order was restored. This was the first time I had found myself using the word 'bubble' to describe my perception of the experience of the person with dementia, for that is how it seemed to me: each person trapped in a glasshouse, seeing only through shadow and distortion, hearing only as through a shell.

This event took place within the context of a research project which explored the place of occupation in the lives of people who have a very advanced dementia (Perrin 1997). The project entailed many hours of observations of severely impaired people, and was carried out in a variety

Box 4.1

Hester is dominating the room with her noise – something like 'ooh wa ow/ beh ow ow/wm ma el we'. It is very loud and accompanied by much circling of the right hand and pointing of the index finger. She looks as though she is laying down the law. Jim comes over, leans over her chair and tries to smack the waving hand. She smacks back and Jim goes away. Elsa on Hester's right is lost in her own repetitive 'My daddy oooh', the my daddy being spoken and the oooh being a long sung note. She is rubbing the fingers of one hand over the fingers of the other. She is in her bubble, but one might imagine that she is making her own noise in competition with Hester – if she mutters and ooohs, she might be able to block out Hester's noise. Marion, two chairs away from Hester, now starts her own special noise, a guttural sound from deep within her throat, as though someone has just stabbed her and she is about to expire. Her gaze ranges around the room, occasionally passing over me sitting near her on the floor, but not engaging. Opposite, David is lying across a recliner chair. His legs are hanging over one arm with feet resting on the floor. His head, over the other arm, has been supported on two pillows on a dining chair. He is alternately twitching and roaring, and from time to time appears to be rather inefficiently trying to masturbate. The TV is on – nobody is looking at it. Lily is slumped in a chair between Marion and Hester. She is not talking or noise-making. She wipes her nose on her cardigan front. Arthur wanders in and wanders out again. Marion's noise gets louder and more dramatic. She sounds as though she is being slowly strangled. It is a cacophony of noise. I am reminded of a zoo, but it is not like a zoo. The noises are not animal noises. Nobody is hearing anybody else. Each is trapped in their own world – their own bubble. Margaret must surely have a terribly sore throat by now. Elsa has stopped. She just sits and stares and occasionally rubs her fingers. Jim wanders in again – no shoes, a large hole in the heel of one sock, both name labels on the outside for all to be able to discover who he is. This is supposed to be the quiet room.

of different residential settings. Some of the research findings were what might have been expected by anyone familiar with the general poverty of occupation that often exists in such settings; for example, many people in residential settings spend the greater portion of their waking day unoccupied; most people respond very positively to occupation. But there were some surprises, some very thought-provoking outcomes. We want to cite two of these outcomes in the context of this discussion on the significance of the carer to the person with dementia.

'Bubble' was the image that came to mind again as I processed the empirical data of the formal research project. In the preliminary phase, I had used dementia care mapping (Kitwood & Bredin 1992) to measure occupation and wellbeing across nine different dementia care settings, and one exercise in the data processing was to compare the overall wellbeing scores of the different units. Results were not as expected. The unit which was dark, cramped, crowded, incessantly noisy and deeply permeated by what Kitwood (1997) would call a 'malignant social psychology' actually had a higher group wellbeing score than the unit which was quiet, spacious, tastefully decorated, and where the overall pattern of care was consistently sensitive and respectful. Similarly, the cavernous, bland Victorian hospital ward at full capacity, had the same group wellbeing score as the newly built, beautifully designed home where the few residents were accommodated in small family-style sitting rooms. This seemed at first very puzzling – I had no doubt about which environments made *me* feel better (or worse) as I sat in them recording my observations over many months. Why would a person with dementia not feel the same? Well, I have wondered if these data are an indication that the immediate environment may have considerably less impact upon severely impaired people than is commonly imagined. Where most of us attach considerable importance to decor, furnishings and congenial company, and where inspection and registration units set standards on room size, equipment for disability and staffing levels, it is actually unclear how much influence many of these things really have on the well-/ill-being of persons who are well advanced in their dementia.

For the unimpaired person, in the doctor's waiting room for example, there is likely to be an acute awareness of her environment, whether or not it impinges upon her conscious thought. She will have an appreciation of whether it is crowded or full, light or gloomy, of the decor and furniture, of health promotion posters on the walls. She will be conscious of the comings and goings of patients, and will probably eavesdrop on conversations around the room. If she is kept waiting long enough, she may discover the number of stripes on the wallpaper or the damp patch on the ceiling, or she may choose to extend her environment by looking out of the window. We suspect that this is not the case with the severely impaired person. For such a person, it seems rather as though the environment has 'shrunk' to envelop her in a kind of glass bubble, which in most cases is about 3 to 4 feet in diameter; that from inside this bubble, the physical conditions of the general environment, along with the conversations and interactions of everyday social intercourse, are perceived in a distorted and muffled fashion and therefore fail to impinge appropriately upon the individual within. What seems to be critical for the client, is what goes on *within* the bubble, within those inches of personal space, and this demands a different concept of 'environment' on our part, if we are to discover and utilise those approaches which can substantially engage the person inside.

The main body of the research alluded to above measured the wellbeing of severely impaired persons in the context of a range of sensorimotor occupations. There were again some very interesting results. Not only did the greater number of observations testify to the overriding importance of the carer's presence in the context of the occupation (in fact only two subjects were able to engage in *any* measure without a carer), but a small number of subjects were so intensively engaged in the personal interaction with the carer delivering the occupation, that they were quite unable to engage with the occupation itself. Why should this be? Is it possible that the greater the impairment, the closer the bubble shrinks to enclose the person inside?

Drama therapist Paula Crimmens (conference address, 1996) has suggested that most human interactions between healthy persons might be represented schematically as shown in Figure 4.1. For a fruitful interpersonal transaction to take place, each party will move towards the other in a measure of some equivalence. New acquaintances will exchange views on the weather and the state of the nation, perhaps share a bus seat or a cup of tea, and relationship is developed. Old friends will share hopes and plans and precious time, and relationship is strengthened and extended. The person with dementia, however (and this may be equally true of persons with other psychological difficulties), has increasing problems as the condition progresses, in making that move outwards toward the other in equal measure. What then occurs, as shown in Figure 4.2 is a fracturing of relationship. Person A has made the usual move of social contact towards person B, but person B's dementia has now got a little more hold than it had when they last met, and B is no longer able to reciprocate. While both parties hold such a position, the fracture is sustained, the gap is not bridged, and there is no meeting point.

In the case described in Box 4.2, there was as yet, certainly no shortage of communication between Harry and Joan – in fact, they were arguing far more than they ever used to. There always seemed to be something to squabble about; nobody could accuse them of not communicating. But there was no *meeting*, and there is a subtle difference. Harry had changed. He no longer thought very much about how he looked, he just wanted to be comfortable. Nor was he able to concern himself with Joan's embarrassment and shame, he could only feel her anger. Harry was no longer able to move out towards Joan as he once would. Joan, for reasons of her

Figure 4.1 Healthy relationship.

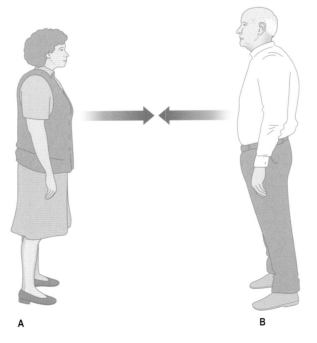

A   B

Figure 4.2   Fractured
relationship.

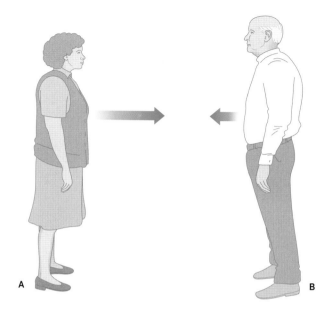

A   B

Box 4.2

Harry had had dementia for about 3 years. He had been a smart man all his
life; he had a military bearing, and was always immaculately dressed. But over
the last year, his wife Joan felt that he had begun to neglect himself. There
were three things that she found difficult. The first was that Harry no longer
seemed to be bothered about wearing a tie; but he had always worn a tie, even
in casual dress, and Joan felt that he should continue to do so. It was important
to keep things as normal as possible, and she felt uncomfortable that he should
be seen without. The second thing that rankled was that he had started to
slouch and shuffle; gone was the upright demeanour and firm step. Although
it was hard to admit, he looked untidy and sloppy, as though he'd given up and
couldn't be bothered any more. And perhaps the most difficult thing was that
he, a man of impeccable manners, was starting to mess with his food. He ate
slowly and fiddled with the contents of his plate. Food would often end up on
the table or on the floor or down his front. It sometimes made her feel sick.

   Joan brought some of her distress and discomfort to the carer's group,
describing the effort she was going to, to hang on to the old Harry. She would
insist upon his wearing a tie, and would usually put it on and tie it for him;
she had constantly to be chivvying him to stand up straight and walk properly
like he used to, and it seemed that she had to have a cloth permanently in
her hand at mealtimes, for she couldn't bear all the spills and splodges. The
most distressing thing though, was all the rows they were now having. Harry
shouted at her and called her an interfering old cow; he had even once or
twice lifted his hand towards her, something he had never ever done in all
their years of marriage. She just couldn't understand why dementia should
make a person so angry.

own interior pain and resistance, was unable to move any further towards Harry. An impasse had been reached; there was no meeting, just a yawning chasm which was threatening to grow ever wider.

Friends in the carer's group were very concerned about this situation. Joan had begun to fear for her own safety, and her friends thought privately that she was quite justified in doing so. But they also saw what Joan herself seemed unable to see, that it was her failure to accept and adapt to the change in Harry that was actually at the root of the arguments and conflict. Because of his cognitive impairments, Harry couldn't change or move. Resolution in any measure, would have to come through Joan, and it would mean having to adopt a position such as that shown in Figure 4.3. Each retreat by Harry would require a further advance by Joan if true meeting was to be sustained over the course of his dementia. The effort and sacrifice and self-denial would have to be all hers. As it turned out, Harry died before his dementia got very much worse, and it was generally felt that perhaps this was the best thing, for Joan seemed unable to move very far at all. It had nothing to do with love or compassion or commitment, for Joan had these in abundance. But somewhere within, there was some fear and damage and despair of her own, which held her back from being able to accommodate herself to her husband's greater needs.

The case in Box 4.3 amplifies further the issue of 'different worlds'. What Joan had been unable to do for Harry, and the careworker for Audrey, Julie *was* able to do. Between Joan and Harry, and careworker and Audrey, there was a communication gap – each was interacting with the other, but there was no meeting. Joan was unable to understand the change in Harry, or his inability to be to her what he once was, and she

Figure 4.3 Restored relationship.

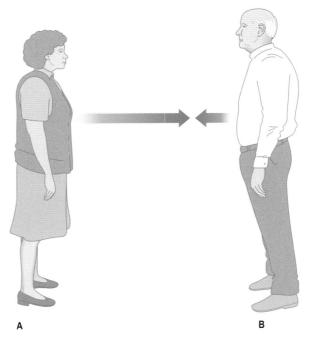

A   B

Box 4.3

It was mealtime in the home, and Audrey was wheeled into the lounge. Audrey has severe dementia, her hands are contracted and her speech is very limited. She can say only a few phrases (like 'Go to bed', 'I love you' and a few swear words) which she repeats in the same loud flat tone over and over. Audrey also has very bright blue, large, expressive, beautiful eyes. The care assistant charged with the task of feeding her pulled over a low stool with one hand, Audrey's dinner in the other (a soft warm mass of splodge). She placed the stool at Audrey's side but then sat facing the opposite direction – her left shoulder almost touching Audrey's left shoulder. She placed the bowl of splodge on her lap, and started to put spoonfuls into Audrey's mouth – all the while looking out of the window. Audrey's eyes tracked left, right, left, right – looking for a face to hook herself into. But there wasn't one, just more faceless spoonfuls of food arriving out of nowhere into her mouth. When she had finished, the careworker stood up, stood over Audrey and wiped her mouth – still with no eye contact, and Audrey's eyes scanning her face. Later that afternoon when a new shift was on duty, a young carer named Julie walked into the day room. She had bright blonde dyed hair, an earring in her nose, lots of earrings in her ears, a black miniskirt, thick black tights and large clumpy Doc Martens on her feet. She had a spouted cup in her hand with, I presumed, tea in it. She pulled the low stool up next to Audrey, and sat astride it so that her face was right up close to Audrey's face. Audrey beamed as her eyes hooked in with Julie's. Both women were twinkling at each other. Without any words, Julie slowly and gently fed Audrey sips of tea, eyes still locked together and smiling, beaming, deeply communicating. She stroked Audrey's face every so often, and Audrey nuzzled in for more. Julie was new, she hadn't any training and she didn't know that she was keeping Audrey in the world for a little longer.

couldn't bridge the gap; they remained estranged and at loggerheads. The careworker either couldn't, or didn't want to understand that there was still a person inside Audrey, able to feel and understand and respond; they remained alienated. Julie however, who in terms of age and culture was a million miles distant from Audrey, did understand. She was able to accept Audrey as she was, unconditionally. She knew that Audrey had no ability to come to her, so she went to Audrey. She crossed the gap – by appreciating Audrey's needs, and adapting her own expectations and actions accordingly. She had established a point of meeting, and harmony of relationship was the result.

The matter which has been particularly concerning us in this chapter, has been (in the Piagetian terminology of Chapter 3) the increasing egocentricity of the person with dementia as the condition advances. Perhaps we should just say a word here about the term egocentricity, for it is important to appreciate that Piaget does not use it with any moral connotation in mind. There is no suggestion here of self-aggrandisement or selfishness, although of course the latter may well feature in a dementia. The term simply refers to a self-centring. We find it helpful to understand the term not so much as an active, voluntary or conscious withdrawal from the environment, but simply as a failure to perceive a progressively narrowing environmental field. We could picture it schematically as shown in Figure 4.4. The person with dementia will first lose sight of A, his wider environment; this might be the wider environs of the town where he lives, or perhaps distant friends or relatives that he sees only from time to time, or possibly peripheral projects that are not particularly meaningful. As his dementia advances, there will come a point where he fails to perceive B as well as A; this could be the layout of his son's house, his new-born grand-daughter, or the model railway he was building in the spare room. Later he will be unable to appreciate A, B *and* C; he will get lost in his own house, fail to recognise his Bowls Club friends, be unable to attempt the daily paper crossword. And so on. We would not therefore perceive this increasing egocentricity as purely a turning-in on oneself; rather, that the external world for the dementing person is changing, and is in a very real sense shrinking.

To perceive the phenomenon in such a way lends further credibility to the 'bubble' and 'meeting' concepts explored above. For if A, B, C and D no longer exist in any significant way for the person with dementia, he is indeed encased in a sort of glass shell, and can only operate within its confines. Research has yet to demonstrate the possibility of 'rementia', which in this analogy would be perceived as a moving from the inner to the outer zones, D to C to B to A. Whilst we hope and certainly work towards such an ideal, the fact remains that if somebody is living in a diminished world of C and D, that is our starting-point, that is where we are going to have to go to meet with him. Trying to reach him from a point somewhere

Figure 4.4 The developing egocentricity of dementia.

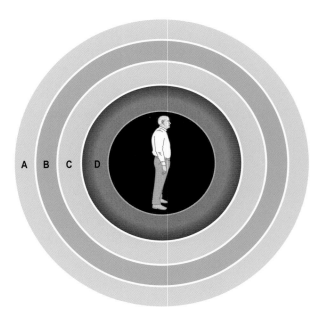

in A or B is quite futile; he cannot cross over towards us, we have to move into his world.

What then does all this mean in practice for those of us who are carers of people who have dementia? How can we sustain that point of meeting in order to be able to engage a person, in order to be able to apply our therapies? We need first to revisit the 'return to childhood' analogy of Chapter 3.

We have proposed that when a person's dementia has advanced to the point where he is experiencing the world primarily in terms of his sensorimotor and reflex faculties, he has the same capacity for operating in the world as very young children. We intend to pursue this metaphor, and there seems to be considerable potential in child care for illumination. Child care does, after all, have a long history of research and development, and it seems unwise to ignore this if there is any chance that it might shed light on the problems of dementia care. We would want to propose that the next question to be considered in this context, is that of a parenting role for carers.

The research alluded to above (Perrin 1997) clearly demonstrated the critical importance of the carer to the wellbeing of the severely impaired person: that such a person is not able to engage in occupations without the intervention of another, and that high levels of wellbeing can be experienced in the context of occupation with another. The overwhelming importance of closeness, of constancy, of playfulness, of physical contact, of eye contact, was the most significant feature of the interventions carried out with the research subjects. As one peruses the literature on attachment between infants and their parents, one can only be struck by the parallels and analogies, and hence the possibilities. Why should not that which is so vital at an early stage of life have some resonance at every stage of life, including the last?

Shaffer (1989) has commented upon the agreement which exists between some of the foremost developmental theorists of our time (Freud, Bowlby, Erikson), on the absolute necessity for healthy development of a stable emotional bond between infant and caregiver. The seminal work on attachment was developed by John Bowlby, who used it as a way of conceptualising the propensity of human beings to make strong affectional bonds to particular others (Bowlby 1977). He was particularly interested in the bond between parent and child, and in the developmental sequelae of disruption to that bond in early childhood (Bowlby 1969, 1973, 1980). The follow-up work of Ainsworth et al (1978) was of considerable influence in furthering the development of attachment theory. Ainsworth et al developed a mechanism for studying attachment behaviour: the 'Strange Situation Test'. This is an assessment procedure in which it is possible to study the responses of children to their parents in unfamiliar situations. The principal finding of their studies using the test was that infants invariably respond in one of three ways: secure, insecure avoidant or insecure ambivalent. Secure infants demonstrate exploratory behaviour in the presence of the parent, distress on separation, and warmth and affection on reunion. The insecure avoidant child shows little interest in exploration whilst with the parent, little distress on separation, and indifference or avoidance of contact on reunion. The insecure ambivalent child shows anxiety and little exploration in the presence of the parent, considerable distress on separation, and ambivalence on reunion, clinging and angry/resentful at the same time.

Recent years have seen a blossoming of interest in the possibility that these attachment patterns of childhood are a useful model for relationships right across the life span (Main et al 1985, Hazan & Shaver 1987, Bartholomew & Horowitz 1991). Bère Miesen (1992) has understood attachment as an explicatory theory for the distressing 'parental fixation' often accompanying dementia. That which Miesen refers to as parent fixation is the outward expression of parent-related needs on the part of the person with dementia. This might take the form of a request to go home or to see a mother or father; an attempt to return home or to find a parent; to perceive himself as back in the family setting, or as being under the threat of parental authority.

Miesen wondered what was at the root of such behaviour, and suggested that it could be related to a number of things: it could be the prevalence of long-term memories in the context of short-term memory loss; it could be part of a reminiscence process about good times; it could be a manifestation of unresolved conflict with parents. Miesen constructed a research procedure called the Standard Visiting Procedure, which was closely allied to the Strange Situation Test, but adapted for use with elderly people and their relatives. He studied 40 persons with dementia and their responses to relatives in unfamiliar situations, and came to the conclusion that parental fixation in dementing people is an expression of their need for safety and security, that the dementing process itself is a 'strange situation' which gradually becomes permanent.

> 'If the bond with the outside world disappears through memory dysfunction, then the demented person will search for some kind of a "hold". But it is precisely these memory dysfunctions which erode feelings of safety and security, because durable affective bonds are not obtainable. This means that the demented elderly person is caught up in a situation that is comparable to a bereavement process which can never be resolved. A vicious circle begins. The exposed needs for safety and security can never be fulfilled. Dementia activates attachment behaviour but at the same time ensures that old and new attachment figures will not remain present in the social environment of the demented person.'

Miesen suggests that in late dementia, parental fixation functions as a form of attachment behaviour, an attempt of the individual to meet his own security and safety needs. He proposes the interesting notion of 'adoption' (with all its connotations of parental care) as a carer's means of responding appropriately to that individual (Miesen 1999).

We would want to propose that behaviours perceived as parent seeking, or indeed, behaviours perceived as childlike in any other fashion, should be responded to by carers in a parental fashion. There is growing support for such a proposal. Häggström & Norberg's (1996) study of carers in a well-respected group-living facility for people with dementia, found a care process set very much in the context of 'family' and governed by an approach which they described as maternal love, thinking and practice. As far as we can determine, these authors are the first to propose 'mothering' as a metaphor for the care of severely impaired people. It is a metaphor, we believe, which has much to offer the future of dementia care, and we will discuss this further in Chapter 10.

Before proceeding, it is perhaps necessary to say something about the acceptability of the term 'mothering' in these days of political correctness. Parenting is probably a less inflammatory term, yet parenting has connotations of control and demand, of authoritarianism; perhaps this a legacy of transactional analysis. Mothering, with its traditional implications of soothing, comforting, holding and nurturing is our preferred term for use in this context. This is not to imply in any way that men are not capable of mothering; we simply find ourselves in agreement with Lamb (1981) that men and women tend to respond to children in different ways, fathers taking more of a playmate role, providing playful physical stimulation and unusual, unpredictable games. (It could perhaps even be suggested that fathering is a model for an earlier stage of dementia, when new and varied playful experiences are especially apposite.) Lamb has noted that when they are distressed or afraid, infants often prefer the company of mother rather than father, and it is this particular quality in mothering which we would want to affirm by use of the term in this context.

Ainsworth's work on the quality of attachments has given rise to the suggestion that caregivers are the 'architects' of the quality of attachments (Shaffer 1989); that attachment, non-attachment or disordered attachment with the one cared for lies in the hands of the caregiver. A caregiver may of course be of either sex, but in fact all of Ainsworth's work was carried out with mothers, presumably a reflection of the times. She drew three pictures of caregiving, suggesting that carers commonly fell into one category:

- Securely attached infants had mothers who were highly sensitive to their signals, who were emotionally expressive, enjoyed close contact, and were likely to encourage exploration.
- Insecure ambivalent infants had mothers whose responses to their child were inconsistent; their responding was often more dependent upon their own emotional state than upon the child's. These mothers were usually interested in their babies, and willing to provide physical contact, but often misinterpreted signals and failed to establish routines.
- Insecure avoidant children had mothers whose style of responding tended to be negative and rejecting. They were unresponsive to the child's signals, and kept physical contact to a minimum; they often showed resentment to the child's interference in their own plans and wishes.

Building on Ainsworth's study, further work has demonstrated that it is not the maternal relationship per se that bestows secure attachment, but the qualities inherent in the mothering. Work with preschool children and their alternative caregivers in day-care facilities (Anderson et al 1981,

Phillips et al 1987) has shown that secure attachments can take place with anyone, provided that certain criteria are fulfilled:

■ there should be a reasonable child to caregiver ratio (4–12:1)
■ caregivers should be warm, emotionally expressive and responsive to bids for attention
■ there should be low staff turnover
■ there should be age appropriate games and activities
■ caregivers should be willing to confer with relatives.

All this has considerable resonance with the dementia carer who is able to appreciate a validity in the mother/child metaphor. We would want to suggest that appropriate care for the person who has dementia should have secure attachment as its focus, and adopt those principles outlined above, namely:

■ carers should be easily accessible, and responsive to clients' signals and bids for attention
■ carers need to be able and free to express emotions in an overt manner
■ carers should enjoy and actively solicit close physical contact with their clients
■ carers should encourage their clients' exploration of and engagement with the immediate environment
■ balanced care should be able to alternate soothing, holding and comforting, with playful, novel stimulation, as indicated by the client's behavioural signals
■ care should aim at consistency of long-term relationship as far as possible with in the constraints of the institutional setting.

It may be, too, that we should understand the behaviour problems commonly observed in residential dementia settings as disorders or failures of attachment. That withdrawal, lack of engagement, clinging, searching, anxiety, fear and challenging responses might be features of disordered attachment would seem to be a proposition worthy of further investigation. If we, as caregivers, are the architects of attachment with our clients, then we must accept responsibility for failing to provide for our clients an environment of sufficiently nurturing relationships.

Such a responsibility puts considerable pressure upon the caring team to ensure accessibility and consistency of response. We cannot necessarily expect Mary to remember that she had a hug and a cuddle half-an-hour ago, or assume that the effects of that hug and cuddle should necessarily last, and satisfy her for the rest of the morning. Perhaps we are going to have to acknowledge that effective care in a dementia setting means always being available, always being ready to affirm and reaffirm relationship, regardless of whether or not a person will be able to receive and use our offering.

Miesen (1999) has proposed the concept of 'adoption' as a consideration regarding the nature of the relationship that we should foster with the person in our care. This is an idea we have found helpful and have discussed further recently (Perrin & Cornes 2007). Adoption is, almost by definition, surrogate mother/fatherhood. It is not about being a friend, even a good friend, nor about being a carer or an advocate, although it may embrace all these facets of relationship. Adoption is a formal and life-long commitment; it is a conscious choice (indeed that is the root meaning of the word) to enter into a relationship and to accept responsibility for another. It assumes above all things a constancy and security of attachment. We believe that it offers a positive working model of relationship for either professional or family carer.

In sum then, we understand childhood and early development to take place in the context of a gradual separation between mother and child, as the child's needs change and skills multiply. In dementia, we might recognise that as skills diminish and dependence grows, there is an increasing need for 'reunion' between mother (-figure) and the impaired person. There are, of course, significant implications of such a proposal for care settings where time constraints and staff shortages often appear to be endemic, and where authorities are struggling to know how to advise their employees where intimacy of relationship and close physical contact are concerned. These are matters which must be addressed if excellence in quality of care is truly our aim.

Chapter 5 continues to deal with the matter of approach, of the therapeutic relationship, but from a slightly different angle – that of the playful practitioner.

Key Points

- Preliminary research suggests that the physical environment may have considerably less impact upon severely impaired people than is commonly imagined.
- The critical physical environment for the person with dementia might be perceived as a bubble – a few feet of personal space, of which he or she is at the centre.
- This idea seems compatible with Piaget's description of egocentricity in the child's preoperational stage of development.
- Empirical research and naturalistic observations by the authors in the clinical setting testify to the overriding importance of the carer's presence to the wellbeing of the person with dementia – closeness, constancy, playfulness, physical contact and eye contact feature as the most important manifestation of effective intervention.
- Carers with a capacity to bring these qualities to the dementia care setting are likely to be able to enter into a person's 'bubble', and can have a profound impact on the wellbeing of the person they care for.
- There is increasing interest in the possibility that the attachment patterns of childhood provide a useful model for relationship right across the life span, and attachment theory has much to offer the field of dementia care.
- Parental fixation may be at the root of commonly observed attachment behaviour in people who have dementia, and 'good mothering' is a quality we should be fostering in dementia carers.

References

Ainsworth M, Blehar M, Waters E, Wall S 1978 Patterns of attachment: a psychological study of the strange situation. Erlbaum, Hillsdale, NJ

Anderson C, Nagle R, Roberts W, Smith J 1981 Attachment to substitute caregivers as a function of center quality and caregiver involvement. Child Development 52:53–61

Bartholomew K, Horowitz L 1991 Attachment styles among young adults: a test of a four category model. Journal of Personality and Social Psychology 61:226–244

Bowlby J 1969 Attachment and loss: Vol 1: Attachment. Hogarth Press, London

Bowlby J 1973 Attachment and loss: Vol 2: Separation. Hogarth Press, London

Bowlby J 1977 The making and breaking of affectional bonds. British Journal of Psychiatry 130:201–210

Bowlby J 1980 Attachment and loss: Vol 3: Loss. Hogarth Press, London

Häggström T, Norberg A 1996 Maternal thinking in dementia care. Journal of Advanced Nursing 24:431–438

Hazan C, Shaver P 1987 Romantic love conceptualized as an attachment process. Journal of Personality and Social Psychology 52:511–524

Kitwood T 1997 Dementia reconsidered: the person comes first. Open University Press, Buckingham

Kitwood T, Bredin K 1992 A new approach to the evaluation of dementia care. Journal of Advances in Health and Nursing Care 1(5):41–60

Lamb M 1981 The development of father–infant relationships. In: Lamb M (ed) The role of the father in child development. Wiley, New York

Main M, Kaplan N, Cassidy J 1985 Security in infancy, childhood and adulthood: a move to the level of representation. In: Bretherton I, Waters E (eds) Growing points of attachment theory and research. Monographs of the Society for Research in Child Development 50(1–2, Serial No 209):66–104

Miesen B 1992 Attachment theory and dementia. In: Miesen B, Jones G (eds) Caregiving in dementia. Routledge and Kegan Paul, London

Miesen B 1999 Dementia in close-up. Routledge, London

Perrin T 1997 The role and value of occupation in severe dementia. Unpublished PhD thesis, University of Bradford

Perrin T, Cornes L 2007 Well-being and being safe. Alzheimer's Care Today 8(3):199–205

Phillips D, McCartney K, Scarr S 1987 Child care quality and children's social development. Developmental Psychology 23:537–543

Shaffer D 1989 Developmental psychology. Brooks/Cole, California

Chapter 5

The playful practitioner

INTRODUCTION

To talk about play in the context of dementia seems at first rather incongruous, and at face value it seems hard to conceive that play might bear some relation to the process or treatment of dementia. If one perceives the usual life course in a linear fashion, beginning at birth and babyhood, and ending at old age and death, play is commonly construed to be at one end and dementia at the other, which rather begs the question, 'What is the relevance of one to the other?'. There are perhaps two responses to such a conundrum. The first is to argue that play or playfulness is a critical feature of human experience at all ages and stages of development, and that play should therefore be as much an integral part of old age as it should in childhood or mid-life. The second is to give further consideration to the perception of life as a circular, rather than a linear phenomenon, a returning whence we came, rather as we have explored in the preceding two chapters. Both notions are valid.

If play is or should be a feature of experience across the life span, and is not just what is commonly understood as the fun and games of childhood development, what actually is it? and what is its significance in adulthood?

One of the first things we need to appreciate is that many great minds have applied themselves to this question over the centuries, and in most of what has been written there is a notable reluctance to attempt to define play.

Indeed, it is hard to find a consensus of opinion among early writers as to its true nature. Reilly (1974), in occupational therapy's first engagement of any real significance with the matter, picks this up. She describes her own struggles with the enigma as 'defining a cobweb', and her review of the principal theoretical contributions to the subject concludes rather dismissively that:

> '*Only the naïve could believe from reviewing the evidence of the literature, that play is a behaviour having an identifiable nature.*'

Well, we ourselves therefore must subscribe to naïveté, for we believe that it is possible to draw out a common denominator, as it were, from the wide diversity of theories as to the nature and purpose of play. No attempt, however, will be made to define the cobweb. The end point of such an exercise is surely just a bald, utilitarian statement that a cobweb is a fly-trap, and consequently our understanding of its beauty, complexity and integrity as a work of nature is entirely lost to us. The full nature of a cobweb is best brought out by description not by definition, and it may indeed be described most precisely, the respective perceptions of the artist, the architect and the zoologist highlighting this quality and that property until a rich appreciation of the whole is understood. The description that follows is an attempt to shed some light on the essential nature of play.

PLAY IS MOVEMENT

In the light of the above, it is interesting to note that even the Oxford English Dictionary has extreme difficulty defining play, its substantial entry resorting to multiple descriptions and imagery. It does, however, offer a good starting point for an explanation of the subject, suggesting a thread or theme which runs throughout the following discussion. The root words offer two broad slants of understanding, both of which are concerned with motile output. The first is the notion of physical exercise, of free unimpeded movement, of brisk action, in living or non-living things. Ideas which are subsumed under this theme are:

- vigorous bodily action
- dance or display
- clapping of hands
- brisk or light movement
- to gambol or frisk (as new born lambs)
- to flit or flutter (as leaves in the wind)
- to change or alternate rapidly (as colours in iridescence)
- to strike lightly upon (as waves, wind, light)
- to flicker, glitter, ripple, vibrate, sway
- to bubble (as a liquid).

The second shade of meaning also has to do with output and action, but stresses activity designed for amusement or diversion. Under this umbrella come games, sport, jest, musical and dramatic performance – all of which distil the notion of enjoyment, pleasure and delight. These elemental concepts will be commented upon more fully later, but it is perhaps worth noting at this point the common threads of spontaneity and freedom and zest, binding what are, in effect, fairly disparate images.

PLAY IS A LIBERATION

The poet Schiller (1875) is perhaps best known in this sphere for under-writing what has since become known as the surplus energy theory of play. He believed that:

> 'An animal works, when a privation is the motor of its activity, and it plays when the plenitude of force is the motor, when an exuberant life is excited to action.'

Schiller saw play as a type of superabundance, as a means of release for an over-accumulation of energy. This theory has been discussed by many across the years but is no longer popular. More significant are Schiller's ideas on the play *impulse* in man, which he sees as fundamental to the order of life. His view of human nature is that it is essentially bipartite: that persons have a sensuous nature (called the sensuous impulse) which exerts control over physical capacities, and a rational nature which exerts control over psychological capacities. This he called the formative impulse. The two aspects of this dual nature are complementary, but there is a third impulse which serves to unite them, and this is the play impulse. Where the sensuous impulse constrains a person by natural laws, and the forma-tive impulse by laws of reason, the play impulse 'will remove all constraint, and set man free'.

> 'Man plays only when he is in the full sense of the word a human being, and he is a perfect human being only when he plays.' (Miller 1970)

We might do well to consider Schiller's speculations, insofar as they must surely challenge our thinking about the person whose 'formative impulse' is gradually disintegrating within the grip of dementia. Indeed, they beg the question as to whether that uniting force of the play impulse, working in harmony with the sensuous nature, can effect any kind of restraint or remission in the inexorable decline of reason in dementia.

PLAY IS STIMULUS SEEKING

The psychologist Berlyne has written extensively on the matter of play. His writing style is complex and rather turgid, but his key ideas are worthy of inclusion here. He is critical of the hold that the matter of 'response selection' has had upon psychology, particularly through the behaviourist era, and (writing in 1960) he indicated that future research needed to be led not by the question, 'What response will this animal make to this stimulus?' but by the question, 'To which stimulus will this animal respond?'. Berlyne believes that play is all about arousal, and suggests that:

'... the chances of a particular stimulus pattern in the contest for control over behaviour depend, among other properties, on how novel the pattern is, to what extent it arouses or relieves uncertainty, to what extent it arouses or relieves conflict, and how complex it is.'

These qualities of novelty, uncertainty, conflict and complexity arouse the organism's mechanisms for action via investigation, exploration and manipulation. Play is to be seen as stimulus-seeking behaviour. Berlyne (1969) observes that humour and its overt behavioural concomitants (laughter and smiling) are also created by these variables.

PLAY IS CREATIVITY

Morris (1969), from the quite different perspective of the zoologist, has made rather similar observations to those of Berlyne. Morris notes that any species of animal life, human or otherwise, engages in what he describes as a 'stimulus-struggle' which has a clear health/survival function. The object of this struggle is consistently to obtain the optimum amount of stimulation from the environment. For our early ancestors, as indeed for wild animals throughout history, this stimulus-struggle has not been a problem – the very demands of survival imposed sufficient challenge in terms of novelty, uncertainty, conflict or complexity to absorb energies fully. However, modern urban man, as indeed urban (zoo or domesticated) animals, is required less and less to engage in survival activity. Adequate food, water, shelter, health, maternity and child care are all relatively easily obtained, and generally speaking are readily available things we purchase, rather than spend time procuring for ourselves.

Morris notes how the cushioning of this new security in modern man can actually impose conditions of gross under-stimulation, and where such is the case, humans or animals will actively seek out or procure for themselves those situations of novelty, uncertainty, conflict or complexity which will return the stimulus balance to optimum. This may result in the constructive and creative use of leisure time where, for example, the factory worker with a repetitive job turns to the sports field or the artist's easel in his leisure hours, thus enhancing pleasure and developing capacities. But it may equally manifest itself in self- or socially destructive ways. Morris (1964) has clearly documented the latter with regard to the animal kingdom; it requires only minimal experience of the institutional care of humans to be aware that all those features observed by Morris in animals are mirrored to a greater or lesser degree in the men, women and young people who populate our institutions.

Morris ponders the question of what it is that drives some individuals towards a positive handling of the stimulus struggle, and some into a negative response. He compares and contrasts the stimulus struggle of the human adult with the play of children, noting particularly the strength of the child's exploratory urge in the face of almost omnipresent novelty and uncertainty. He proposes that the answer to individual and societal growth and progress lies in the retention of the creative essence of the play of childhood into maturity. What we need, he argues, are 'childlike adults':

> *'The child asks new questions; the adult answers old ones; the childlike adult finds answers to new questions. The child is inventive; the adult is productive; the childlike adult is inventively productive. The child explores his environment; the adult organises it; the childlike adult organises his explorations and, by bringing order to them, strengthens them. He creates.' (Morris 1969)*

Morris is, in effect, expressing Berlyne's stimulus-seeking exploration of novelty and uncertainty in terms of creativity, which he clearly sees as critical to the health and wellbeing of individuals and societies.

THE EXPERIENCE OF RELATIONSHIP

Also understanding play as creativity, yet from a radically different viewpoint of child development, is the paediatrician and child psychiatrist Donald Winnicott. He perceived the play of the child as critical to healthy emotional and social development (Winnicott 1971). He was concerned that play should not be understood purely in the context of the inner, personal, psychic world of subjective experience. He believed that play inhabits a third, intermediate area, and sought to 'locate' it in the hypothetical 'space' between child and mother – specifically, in that potential space occupied by the child's repudiation of the object (mother) as 'not me'. Play, in this sense, facilitates the developmental process in which child and object are first merged; over time, object is repudiated, reaccepted and perceived objectively. Essentially, he perceived play as an essential component for the satisfactory separation of child from mother, the 'not me' from the 'me'.

Winnicott's hypothetical space is the 'playground' where play starts and develops, but it can only function and mature in the context of a relationship of trust and confidence in the reliability of the mother. The child's creative move towards autonomy is nurtured in such a climate, increasingly so as the mother relinquishes her own adaptability to, and identifying with the child's needs. Where there is no constant mother-figure, or where the mother-figure is not a sufficiently reliable presence for the child to gain trust and confidence, emotional development is likely to be impaired.

Our view is that play sustains health. Play facilitates 'safe' separation in our maturational process; it brings about our awareness of 'me' and 'not me', and gives us all we need to be able to form relationships. Without play, our capacity for relationship and sociality are seriously impoverished.

THE FULLEST EXPRESSION OF HUMANITY

It is interesting to note that the essence of some of these themes is echoed in the metaphysical writings of certain theologians – an unexpected vein of wisdom, but one worth tapping.

Like Morris, the priest and academic Romano Guardini (1930) links the play of the child and the creativity of the adult. Like Winnicott, he understands play as the heart of relationship. In his exposition of the Christian liturgy as play, he discourses on the purposelessness of play, implying that its very purpose*less*ness imbues it with meaning*ful*ness:

> '*And because it does not aim at anything in particular, because it streams unbroken and spontaneously forth, its utterance will be harmonious, its form clear and fine; its expression will of itself become picture and dance, rhyme, melody and song. That is what play means; it is life, pouring itself forth without an aim, seizing upon riches from its own abundant store, significant through the fact of its own existence. It will be beautiful too, if left to itself, and if no futile advice or pedagogic attempts at enlightenment foist upon it a host of aims and purposes, thus denaturising it.*' (Guardini 1930)

Guardini is suggesting here that play is the fullest expression of our humanity, and that it is as children at play that we touch the heart of our relationship with God. He appears here to be unfolding the biblical doctrine of needing to become as little children in order to attain to the kingdom of God; only the child truly plays, therefore only the child may realise true relationship with God.

The Catholic theologian Karl Rahner (1972) too, sees play and creativity as essentially the same, their human expression being an attempt to share in the 'Godness' of the creator God. Rahner echoes Guardini's sentiments on purposelessness, understanding God in his act of creation as God the Player (Deus Ludens); the creation was not necessary, 'meaningful but not necessary'. Rahner is concerned not to impute flippancy or triviality to his 'playing' God, rather stressing the opposite. What he particularly wishes to highlight is the freedom personified in Deus Ludens. He was/is free to create what and as he wishes, constrained by nothing and no-one. Creation was no obligation; it was the expression of personal choice motivated by personal desire. For Rahner, God as Deus Ludens gives credence to our understanding of man as Homo Ludens (Huizinga 1949).

FESTIVITY AND FANTASY

Cox (1969) develops the notion of man as Homo Ludens. Cox chronicles the decline of celebration, ritual, myth and vision in the western world, suggesting that something deeply fundamental to the order of life is being lost in the process. Implicit in the notion of man as Homo Ludens, declares Cox, is man as Homo Festivus and Homo Fantasia also. Festivity and fantasy are not just things he does, they are part of the very essence of his being; he *is* a festive and fanciful being. If man turns his back on these external manifestations of his deepest spiritual nature, he places his very survival in grave jeopardy.

Cox defines festivity as the capacity for genuine revelry and joyous celebration, noting how it anchors us in the present by its affirmation of the past. Fantasy is defined as the faculty for envisioning radically alternative life situations, which can enable man to extend the frontiers of the future. Together, festivity and fantasy have the capacity to expand and enhance the experience of the individual and 'help make man a creature who sees himself with an origin and a destiny, not just as an ephemeral bubble'.

Cox points out how recent centuries have repressed man's celebrative and imaginative faculties by their emphasis on man as worker and man as thinker. The eulogising of labour, science, technology and intellectual achievement have consigned festive and fanciful play to the archives of human experience:

> '*Cut a man off from his memories or his visions and he sinks to a depressed state. The same is true for a civilization. So long as it can absorb what has happened to it and move confidently toward what is yet to come its vitality persists. But when a civilization becomes alienated from its past and cynical about its future, as Rome once did, its spiritual energy flags. It stumbles and declines.*'

Such a repression, he suggests, is causing a shrinking psyche and a crumbling spirit. Festive occasions are still paid lip service, but have become hollow and sterile; fantasy is experienced second-hand from the ubiquitous media, stifling innate creativity. The answer lies in a revival of festive occasions which are marked by:

- legitimate excess – 'a kind of social paroxysm in which the more instinctive and disorderly components of human life are temporarily allowed to express themselves'
- celebrative affirmation – 'saying yes to life'
- juxtaposition – a contrast which is 'noticeably different from everyday life'.

Also required is a renewed attention to fantasy, or what Cox describes as advanced imagining, in which we:

> '*... abolish the limits of our powers and perceptions ... give reign ... to physically impossible exploits and even to logically contradictory events.*'

The individual, the society that is able to fantasise is able to stimulate, to innovate, to change; in short it is able to survive.

PLAY IS A DISPOSITION

We have so far examined play largely in the light of its function as an abstract noun, as light and movement, freedom and creativity, festivity and fantasy. But perhaps one of the most helpful ways of studying play is to understand it as an attitude – playfulness. One of the first to remark upon the utility of viewing play as playfulness was the psychologist Millar (1968):

> '*Perhaps play is best used as an adverb; not as a name of a class of activities, nor as distinguished by the accompanying mood, but to describe how and under what conditions an action is performed.*'

The theoretical model of optimal experience developed by Csikszentmihalyi and his colleagues (1975, 1988, 1992) arrives at similar conclusions. He suggests first of all that there needs to be a reassessment of the 'deeply entrenched dichotomy' between work and play; that to think of the two concepts as structurally discrete and mutually exclusive is unhelpful. A more profitable viewpoint from which to study the phenomenon of play is that of experience rather than structure. He notes how attention to structure has directed and confined earlier thinking to the study of games (Huizinga 1949, Caillois 1961), and believes that such constraints impede a full appreciation of the richness of the concept. What is work to one may be play to another, and vice versa; therefore what is important is to understand that the experience of joy, satisfaction and total involvement in life which might be regarded as 'l'esprit de jeu' (the spirit of play) may imbue not only conventionally perceived 'play' activities, but also those more usually construed as work.

Csikszentmihalyi has studied playful behaviour empirically (1975), and determined that its function is to produce that specific 'l'esprit de jeu' state of experience, which he has called 'flow'. Thus the architect may experience flow as much in the design and construction that constitute his working day, as in the dancing that he chooses to engage in in his spare time. Likewise the landscape gardener whose leisure hours are committed to chess playing. From such a perspective, structural differences are artificial; the key is the common experience. Csikszentmihalyi (1975) also observes the play of children, noting the natural, unforced evidence of 'flow' in all they do:

> 'What children do is "play" only by the conventional wisdom of adult perspective. One could say just as well that what they do is work. But both labels are confusing: what children do most of the time is interact with the environment on a level at which their skills match opportunities. Left to themselves, children seek out flow with the inevitability of a natural law. They act without interruption if they can use their bodies, their hands, or their brain to produce feedback which proves that they can control the environment. They stop only when the challenges are exhausted, or when their skills are.'

Csikszentmihalyi suggests that in western society, the spirit of play or flow which is so natural and abundant in children, has largely been 'educated' out of us by young adulthood through a culture and an educational system which eulogises concrete results and extrinsic rewards. Others agree – Eric Berne (1964), one of the fathers of transactional analysis, states:

> 'A little boy sees and hears birds with delight. The "good father" comes along and feels he should "share" the experience and help his son "develop". He says "That is a jay, and this is a sparrow". The moment the little boy is concerned with which is a jay and which is a sparrow, he can no longer see the birds or hear them sing. He has to see and hear them the way his father wants him to. Father has good reason on his side, since few people can afford to go through life listening to the birds sing, and the sooner the little boy starts his "education" the better. Maybe he will be an ornithologist when he grows up.'

From her extensive observations of children at playschool, Crowe (1984) believes that the manipulation of play for educational ends has so trivialised it, that we no longer see or recognise it as part of the life-force itself:

> 'We seem hell-bent on robbing children of their childhood. That magic word "play" is becoming associated with toys or "play situations" structured to encourage linguistic and intellectual development, and my heart goes out to the child who backed away from a wide choice of proffered toys and activities with the telling words "I don't want to do any of those things – couldn't I just play?".'

Csikszentmihalyi's experiments on flow deprivation support his contention that unless adult society learns the critical importance of flow to human experience, and how to ensure that its members encounter it, its future phylogenetic path will be increasingly characterised by escape and over-consumption. Individuals and groups who are unable to build intrinsically-rewarding experiences into their lives will suffer boredom, anxiety or apathy, from which escape can all too often mean the alienation of mental illness, substance abuse, addictions and even crime.

> 'The lack of intrinsic rewards is like an undiscovered virus we carry in our bodies; it maims slowly but surely.' (Csikszentmihalyi 1975)

The future is in the rediscovery and restoration to experience of flow. One way or another, says Csikszentmihalyi, if human evolution is to go on, we shall have to learn to enjoy life more thoroughly.

Also supporting the concept of play as playfulness is the theoretical model of educationalist Lieberman (1977), who through her empirical studies on playfulness in children, adolescents and adults, manages to pull together a number of the aforementioned ideas of play as freedom, as fantasy, as spirit, as creativity. From her direct observations of young children at play, Lieberman catalogued a core of traits that constitute playfulness, and postulated that there is a developmental continuity throughout life, playfulness surviving play and becoming a personality trait in adulthood. She offers a schematic representation to facilitate the expression of her ideas (Fig 5.1), which might be summarised by suggesting that playfulness derives from the inter-relationships between play, imagination and creativity, and expresses itself through sense of humour, spontaneity and manifest joy.

It is also worthy of note that her work in educational settings led Lieberman to remark upon the impact that playful qualities in teachers have in engendering playfulness in students. She argues for the nurturing of the playful spirit in individuals from infancy to old age, believing that the truly playful 'childlike' person has a rich resource of strategy for coping with the vicissitudes of life. She believes that educationalists who seek to foster in their students the playful spirit with all its attendant flexibility, creativity and positive outlook, will have performed an important service to the next generation.

What Lieberman describes as 'playfulness' in the adult is not an uncommon concept, being described by other authors variously under the terms

Figure 5.1 Model of relationships among play, imagination and creativity, and playfulness.

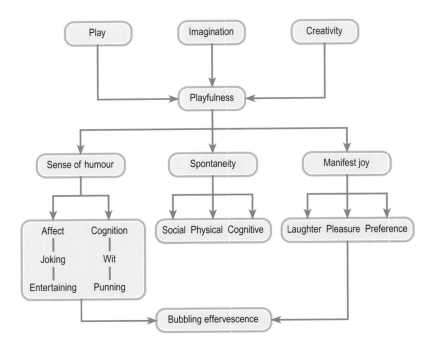

the 'inner child' or 'the child within', and in some cases the 'real' or 'true' self. The inner child is the term preferred in this context. Although Jung introduced the concept (Essays on a Science of Mythology, 1949), it did not find its way into common psychological parlance until the 1960s, in the form of an innovative model of psychotherapy called transactional analysis (TA). TA introduced to the field a standardised vocabulary, language and practice which challenged the esoteric vagaries of psychiatry, making an understanding of interpersonal behaviours available to the lay person.

TA suggests that within each person reside three distinct ego states, which Berne (1961) has called the Parent, the Adult and the Child. The Parent is that set of feelings, attitudes and behaviour patterns belonging to an individual, which are derived from cerebral 'recordings' of everything that person's parents said and did during his childhood. It is in effect the 'taught' aspect of life. The Child is that set of feelings, attitudes and behaviour patterns emanating from 'recordings' of internal events, or the responses of the child to all that he sees, hears and feels. It is in essence the 'felt' aspect of life, the child having no language with which to construct meanings, being dependent on its feelings for understanding and assimilating its experiences of the world. The Adult is that autonomous set of feelings and attitudes and behaviour patterns issuing from the person's ability to find out for himself, to compare and contrast the 'taught' experiences of his Parent, with the 'felt' experiences of his Child. The Adult might be considered a 'thought' or 'data processing' aspect of life. Transactional analysis itself deals with the interplay between these inner states in interpersonal relations.

Developing Berne's original work, Harris (1967) notes the Child's inherent creativity and curiosity, the desire to explore and know, to touch and feel, which expose it to a range of negative feelings to be sure – frustration, anger, loneliness – but for all of which there is a counterpart:

> '... the glorious pristine feelings of first discoveries. In the Child are recorded the countless grand a-ha experiences, the firsts in the life of the small person, ... the first stroking of the soft kitten ... the first submarine chase of the bar of soap, the repetitive going back to do these glorious things again and again.'

It is Harris' contention, however, from his observations of both children and adults, that in the vast majority of us, negative feelings far outweigh the positive. He goes as far as to suggest that everyone has (in the language of TA) a 'not-OK' Child. Writing more recently, Capacchione (1988) picks up this theme, maintaining that by the time most of us reach adult life, our natural, healthy childlike traits are so wounded that they are nearly dead, or at least distorted beyond recognition. Whitfield (1982) is in agreement, identifying a number of environmental factors which might be responsible for this, such as substance abuse, chronic mental or physical illness, child abuse or extreme parental rigidity, perfectionism, punitiveness and inconsistency. Nevertheless, all authors agree that however repressed the inner child, all is not lost, and that a return to health and wholeness is achievable by recognising, identifying and liberating those feeling, intuitive traits that are the childlike part of our selves. We need to play, and in playing there is a restoration of the childhood inheritance that is so rightfully ours.

PLAY IS ENCOUNTER

What we have been attempting to do in preceding chapters is to put together a theoretical construct which is perhaps best understood in the context of *encounter*; for if there is a common denominator running right through the foregoing material, it is that. It seems important at this point to pause and recap, to pull together some of the threads of our discussion.

We first introduced the concept of encounter in Chapter 2, and we saw that encounter is the seat of creativity; that the tension and intensity of encounter, person to person and person to object, is the dynamic of new birth, of the truly creative act. We saw how such an idea was shadowed in the root meanings of the word occupation, and wondered if we weren't maybe talking about two sides of the same coin. We explored how meaning in life is to be found not within our selves alone, but in our relationship and encounter with the world around us.

Health and wellness too, are not to be found in a state of passive ease, but in an encounter, indeed a struggle, with the vicissitudes of the environment in which we find ourselves. We discussed the empirical research which has demonstrated clearly the relation between psychological wellbeing and encounter with the physical and social world of which we are a part.

Permeating this whole discussion was the notion that there is some equivalence between one's level of health and wellbeing and the intensity of one's encounter; in other words, optimum health and wellbeing lie in a full and committed engagement, an engagement of intensity and single-mindedness.

In Chapter 3, we began to pursue the notion of cognitive development and cognitive disintegration in terms of encounter. Through Piaget's developmental theory, we understood the child's increasing intensity of encounter with an ever-expanding world, and we also considered the possibility that the experience of the person with dementia was a 'reversal' of this, as the person's ability to engage with a shrinking world progressively diminishes. The story of Brian portrayed a man whose faculty for encounter with people and places and things was gradually dwindling and distorting, and finally snuffed out altogether.

Chapter 4 pursued this further in the context of encounter and the human relationship. We saw how communication and encounter are not the same thing; one might well experience the first without the second, but never the second without the first. We saw too, how the dementing person's diminishing faculty for encounter can fracture an existing relationship, unless it is met with an increased intensity from the other party. We revisited the 'return to childhood' analogy, and explored the concept of encounter as attachment between child and parent-figure. We proposed the notion that as a dementia advances, the need for deep contact grows; the gradual relinquishing of the parent by the child in early life is mirrored by the developing need for a parent-figure in the dementing person.

In this chapter we have not departed from the theme of encounter, but we have started to look at the potential of *playful* encounter. We have continued with the theme of engagement with the world, but have shifted the focus on effortful striving in action, to notions of spontaneity, freedom and joy, captured so neatly by Lieberman's term 'bubbling effervescence'. We suggested in Chapter 3 that dementia might be understood as a journey, a transition from the world of encounter with places, objects and events, to one of encounter with people; a transition from a world of doing to a world of being. If this is such a journey, and we believe it is, then play is surely an appropriate medium for such a transition to take place. We remember that Winnicott (see p. 75) has actually used the term 'playground' to describe that place which exists between mother and child, where play occurs and is developmentally constructive in the separation process. We propose a similar concept of playground, where playful encounter is a cohesive factor in the 'reunion' of person with dementia and parent-figure.

THE PLAYFUL PRACTITIONER

What does this mean in practice? What is 'playful encounter', and how can it be generated in the clinical setting? Well, first and foremost, there are those fundamental prerequisites of secure attachment that are set out on page 68. But more than that, we believe that there is a certain disposition, a certain personality type, that has a greater facility than most to engage people who have dementia. The person who is able to engage in playful encounter is essentially the person whose own 'inner child' is free and accessible; who is confident and at ease with the way they use their body and voice and emotions; who is spontaneous and immediate, and able intuitively to adopt a stance of openness, unconditional acceptance and receptivity to whatever the person with dementia wishes to bring to the encounter. We have all seen such people in action: the care assistant who notices a tapping foot and turns it into a shared and enjoyable dance; the hairdresser who engages freely and authentically in a rich two-way stream of inconsequential small-talk; the domestic who hears the humming and joins in with her own voice and the rhythm of her dusting. These, we believe, are the qualities of true playfulness; these are the qualities which have real potential to enrich the wellbeing of people with dementia; these are the qualities which attract and engage those whose sense of 'other' and 'out there' is diminishing.

As an interesting addendum, it is worth noting that these qualities are not necessarily common to the average professional. Our concern for the future of dementia care should lie not only in the type and the nature of the occupations we bring, but in the development of those personal attributes in ourselves which will imbue those occupations with the qualities which matter. For some, these qualities are inborn. They are lucky. For others of us they are not. But whether they come naturally or we have to work at them, the degree to which we are able to enrich the occupations we offer with a playful disposition will, we believe, be the yardstick by which we will measure our therapeutic effectiveness as practitioners in dementia care.

Key Points

- Play is a critical feature of health and wellbeing across the life span, not just in childhood.
- Play has at its heart a concept of free, unimpeded movement, liberation.
- One of the most significant manifestations of play is creativity.
- In early developmental terms, play stands as part of the separation process between mother and child.
- In dementia, playful encounter is a cohesive factor in the 'reunion' of the person with dementia and the 'mother'-figure.
- To understand play in terms of structure, i.e. this activity is play and that activity is not play, is unhelpful; what is play to one is work to another.
- Play is better understood as a disposition, i.e. any activity may be made a playful activity by virtue of the qualities we bring to it, either as a participant or as a caregiver.
- Playfulness expresses itself in humour, spontaneity and manifest joy.
- The 'playful practitioner' is a helpful model for the effective dementia carer.

References

Berlyne D 1960 Conflict, arousal and curiosity. McGraw-Hill, New York

Berlyne D 1969 Laughter, humor and play. In: Lindzey G, Aronson E (eds) Handbook of social psychology. Addison-Wesley, New York

Berne E 1961 Transactional analysis in psychotherapy. Grove Press, New York

Berne E 1964 Games people play. Penguin, Harmondsworth

Caillois R 1961 Man, play and games. Free Press, New York

Capacchione L 1988 The power of your other hand. Newcastle, CA

Cox H 1969 Feast of fools. Harvard University Press, Cambridge, MA

Crowe E 1984 Play is a feeling. George Allen and Unwin, London

Csikszentmihalyi M 1975 Beyond boredom and anxiety. Jossey-Bass, California

Csikszentmihalyi M, Csikszentmihalyi I 1988 Optimal experience: psychological studies of flow in consciousness. Cambridge University Press, Cambridge

Csikszentmihalyi M 1992 Flow: the psychology of happiness. Rider, London

Guardini R 1930 The spirit of the liturgy. Sheed and Ward, London

Harris T 1967 I'm OK – you're OK. Pan, London

Huizinga J 1949 Homo Ludens. Routledge and Kegan Paul, London

Jung C, Kerenyi C 1949 Essays on a science of mythology. Bollingen Series, Princeton, NJ

Lieberman J 1977 Playfulness: its relationship to imagination and creativity. Academic Press, New York

Millar S 1968 The psychology of play. Penguin, Harmondsworth

Miller R 1970 Schiller and the ideal of freedom. Clarendon Press, Oxford

Morris D 1964 The response of animals to a restricted environment. Symposium of the Zoological Society of London 13:99–108

Morris D 1969 The human zoo. Cape, London

Rahner K 1972 Man at play. Herder and Herder, New York

Reilly M 1974 Play as exploratory learning. Sage, CA

Schiller F 1875 Essays aesthetical and philosophical. George Bell, London

Whitfield C 1982 Healing the child within. Health Communications, Pompano Beach, FL

Winnicott D 1971 Playing and reality. Tavistock, London

Chapter 6

Principles of good practice in dementia care

As we start to make the all-important move from theory to practice, there are some additional principles that need addressing – principles of good practice which we need to consider as we commence our treatment plan.

PROCESS OR PRODUCT?

The process of engaging in an occupation is more important than its product

Centuries ago, the philosopher Aristotle (Ostwald 1962) had some wise words to say about activity in the human species. He probably didn't have twentieth century occupational therapists in mind as he wrote them, but they are nevertheless pertinent, and worthy of consideration. Aristotle's view of human activity is that it is essentially of two kinds, which he calls *kinesis* and *energeia*. He reckoned that kinesis refers to activities which are goal directed, and gave examples of walking, home-building, weaving, learning. He described kinetic activities as incomplete or imperfect in themselves, insofar as they are only 'completed' when the goal is attained – whether that be a destination, a new house or a length of cloth. Energeia, on the other hand, refers to activities which do not have an end distinct from themselves; the end is inherent in the activity itself. In other words, the activity is done for its own sake. He suggested that energeic activities might include seeing, knowing, living well, and in their 'completeness' are considered 'perfect', superior to kinesis.

Subsumed within this concept of kinesis and energeia is a further differentiation between making and doing. Making is a goal-directed activity in which an agent works upon a malleable entity in order to bring some product into being; it is always a kinetic process. Doing is always energeic (for its own sake), though energeia is in itself a much richer concept, tending towards a sense of actualising latent potential.

We, of course, may not wish to get into an argument about which type of activity is more 'perfect' than the other, but nevertheless the two-fold concept is helpful, and there is an important principle here. For goal-directed activity, the purpose is the end-in-view; the doing of the activity is purposeful only insofar as it works towards achieving its end. It is thus, in a sense, an occupation of the future: 'At such and such a time, I shall achieve such and such a goal'. And being an occupation of future time, it is therefore dependent upon a certain cognitive capacity for satisfactory completion; for example, one must be able to remember what has gone before, apply the appropriate sequence of tasks, hold the goal in view, plan whether to take this route or that, recognise the required conclusion. A fragmented cognition brings about a fragmented 'doing', and can render the goal unachievable; if an integral task or step in that sequence of 'doing' cannot be hooked via memory on to the previous step, or via reason and planning on to the next, it becomes divorced from purpose and has only a life of its own, which may or may not have meaning for that person. An example might illuminate.

Kneading dough is an essential stage in the bread-making process. It is linked to a preparatory stage of mixing yeast with flour, and a succeeding phase of setting the dough in a warm place to rise. Now it may be that a person in early dementia still has an active recall, and a faculty for forward planning. But the more impaired person may well struggle to link any one of those steps with another. After all, a bowl of flour with some putty-coloured liquid in it just looks like a porridgy sludgy mess. There is nothing about it which says 'I am the forerunner of a beautiful, scented, wholemeal loaf – knead me'. Neither is there anything about a solid lump of cold puddingy dough that offers any indication of the risen, round-topped crusty-baked thing it will become. So why should we expect the person to invest any particular meaning or goal in kneading this dough? Such a person is increasingly living 'of the moment', unhooked from what has gone before and unrelated to what will come after. Therefore, surely it is only the experience of that kneading process right now that is important. Only if this activity has a clear impact upon the wellbeing of the person, is it of value as occupational therapy.

We suggested, in Chapter 3, a view that dementia is a journey from a world of doing to a world of being, and recognised the validity of Ignatieff's proposition that for the person in late dementia there is only now, this instant, the way the ice cream tastes when it is on your tongue.

This, we feel, is the key to the superiority of process over product in dementia care. Process is now, of the present moment; product is some time, of the future. Therefore, process is what is of particular importance to the person with dementia; product might ultimately hold some meaning for a person, but the therapeutic stance should not demand it. If Arthur is pummelling dough with every sign of pleasure and satisfaction, the outcome is immaterial. It is unlikely that he will associate the arrival of a fresh baked loaf two hours later as anything to do with himself anyway.

None of this is intended in any way to diminish the place of goal-directed activity in the therapeutic programmme. Rather, it is to set it in its appropriate context. We will see in Chapter 8 that such activity is the common currency of the unimpaired person, and it may therefore be used entirely appropriately in the earlier stages of dementia. But we need to bear in mind that the capacity of most of our clients for 'doing' is diminishing, and we need to assist them to accommodate this change in a gradual relinquishing of end-products and goals, and an embracing of the 'here and now' experience.

The product of the Tea Group described in Box 6.1, was unimportant; in fact it turned into a rather sticky and messy affair, but that did not matter to Dermott, and it did not matter to me either. It was the process of connecting, or engaging in the context of a shared activity that was important for both of us. We ate together, laughed together, had fun together, but most important of all, Dermott held the power. We believe that Dermott's sustained and committed engagement with this activity was a clear indication that right now, for him, this was a rewarding, meaningful, and hence therapeutic experience.

Box 6.1

Dermott is a fit, agile man, still very young compared with most of the people who come into the ward for day care sessions. Dermott is actually very damaged, far more so than he looks; this is in part because of his youthfulness and physical fitness, and also because he is very funny, well able to crack jokes and cover things up quickly and easily. But in fact, Dermott cannot unwrap a sweet and put it into his mouth. He gets confused about which is the wrapper and which is the sweet; he has a real problem differentiating between objects generally. He is unable to recognise objects for their purpose, and he cannot therefore do even very simple daily living tasks. I invited him to the Tea Group today, knowing that someone would have to support him and compensate for his difficulty, so that he could remain an integral part of the group. I sat next to him, and offered him the bread which he wanted. He was not able to butter his bread, to lift the knife and put the knife in the butter to spread on his bread, or to put jam on the bread. But once I had spooned some jam on to the bread he was able to spread some of it, although the next thing he did was to dip his knife into the tea and try to spread that on! But we got through. We found our way into a sort of routine, so that at each stage of the sequence I would ask whether he wanted to do it, or whether he wanted me to do it, and we got into a banter and a joke about it so that, although he clearly wanted me to do it, he nevertheless remained very much in control, and led the way through the activity. This was precisely what we had wanted to achieve by this group session. Dermott does not normally sit down for longer than 30 seconds; even in the exercise group he often prefers to stand or to wander around. Certainly that is what he does in the absence of anything concrete to focus upon. But today he sat and stayed for the whole group session, which lasted on this occasion for approximately 40 minutes.

COGNITIVE OR SENSORY?

Cognitive approaches should be used with caution in dementia care

Many of the activities that we use in dementia care have a strong cognitive component: for example, reality orientation, the quiz, the discussion, following a recipe, a game of cards, etc. To be able satisfactorily to engage with such an activity requires a certain cognitive capacity. One must remember what has gone before, plan what is to come, understand the ultimate goal, appreciate the relevance of the rules, communicate with other parties, and so on. An impairment in any of these faculties can disrupt successful engagement with the activity, and can render a person unable to some degree to carry out the activity as they once would.

Diminished performance in our client may or may not trouble us unduly (we are all well used to impairment and disability), but how sure are we that it is not troubling that person? We believe that people with dementia retain at least some measure of insight into their degenerating condition, if not throughout, at least until the latter stages of decline, and if diminished wellbeing results then this cannot be called therapy. We also believe that many of the challenging behaviours that we meet in dementia care are but the product of that insight – the rage, frustration and anguish of knowing that you can't be and do as you once could. Therefore, to inflict upon somebody an activity which he can no longer carry out with the same finesse that he once could is tantamount to setting him up for failure, and has the potential for being damaging in the extreme. It might not, but it might – and that is always our dilemma.

Have you ever played Trivial Pursuit? Great fun if you have a wide-ranging general knowledge and can shine; not so much fun if you haven't. If you haven't, you can often get away with playing in groups and hiding in the context of a team. But if you are playing for yourself, everything that you know (and don't know) is exposed for all to see. Knowledge of one's own deficit can be stressful, and induce shame and withdrawal; and that goes as much for the unimpaired person as for the person with dementia. If we can feel bad in a trivial game of Trivial Pursuit, how much more might our dementing client?

However, one might argue from the 'use it or lose it' point of view. We had a letter a while ago from a gentleman who found himself as the main carer of a friend with dementia. Out of concern to maintain her at as high a level of functioning as possible, he was writing to ask if his approach to her 'therapy' was a profitable one. This gentleman was a retired academic, and was bringing something of this background to the therapeutic programme that he had set up for her. The programme was a series of mental exercises that comprised numbering sequences backwards and forwards, simple sums, word sequences and word games. He felt that to take her regularly and frequently through these exercises might help to maintain cognitive function. He was in fact operating from a point of view that perceives the brain as a muscle requiring exercise. There is indeed some evidence that disuse or understimulation of cognitive faculties leads to further impairment (Diamond 1976, 1978), but the 'muscle and exercise' analogy is rather a suspect one and should be treated with caution. For

Box 6.2

Elsa, the lady referred to in Box 4.1, had very little language left, just a few odd stereotyped phrases. Mostly she just sat quietly in her chair, unresponsive to events in the environment around her; but she did have an habitual 'My daddy oooh', said and sung in long periods of repetitive vacuum. She would often though, engage readily in conversation (much of which was of the non-verbal kind) when staff had time for her. On one occasion, when she was looking rather down and depressed, a very chatty member of staff went to sit with her and attempted to engage her in conversation. She talked of this and that, inconsequential things, and wasn't bothered by Elsa's lack of response. But Elsa was starting to look panicky; it looked as though she was desperately trying to stay in touch with this stream of chatter, while actually being radically outpaced. Suddenly she lifted her head and uttered a loud, sustained trilling noise, which stopped all members of staff on the unit dead in their tracks. Everyone was very used to 'My daddy oooh', and largely ignored it, but nobody had ever heard this before. We are unlikely ever to know what was at the root of it, but it is hard to understand it as anything other than a response to extreme overstimulation.

every piece of research that promotes cognitive challenge as a means to improving function and wellbeing (Greene et al 1979, 1983, Hanley et al 1981), there is another advocating reduced stimulus (Cleary et al 1988, Hall 1994); this latter proposition is supported in fact by the reaction of Elsa in Box 6.2.

The key surely must lie in finding a balance, and this was our response to the gentleman who wrote to us. Our critical task is to monitor closely the impact of the activity upon the wellbeing of the person to whom we are delivering it. If the activity is being received with outward evidence of pleasure and satisfaction, then we have good grounds for proceeding. If the activity is clearly generating anxiety and distress, or if there are attempts at avoidance, we may be fairly sure that it is neither helpful nor constructive. This is person-centered care; we look for the client to lead *us* into an understanding of what is good and right for them. The aerobics teacher may insist 'no pain, no gain'; we have no such remit.

We must therefore handle cognitive activities very carefully in dementia care. We are on safer ground with activities that have a strong sensorimotor component. We know that sensorimotor faculties are retained generally much longer than cognitive faculties, and there is an extensive literature demonstrating the adverse physical and psychological effects of sensory deprivation, and affirming the need for optimum levels of sensory stimulation in the human environment (Bexton et al 1954, Bower 1967). There is also a growing consensus of empirical evidence amongst practitioners that the sensory pathway is the prime route to effective communication and wellbeing in dementia (Birchmore & Clague 1983, Paire & Karney 1984, Rogers et al 1987, Perrin 1997a).

RELAXATION OR AROUSAL?

Which is the focus of treatment?

Related in some respects to the above matter of a sensory approach to activity, is the question of relaxation or arousal as a therapeutic focus. Which is it that we seek in our intervention? Does it matter? We think it does.

Sometimes the task is very clear: for the person who has become withdrawn and lethargic through institutional routine and neglect, we use occupation to arouse and stimulate, to challenge and quicken; for the person upset and distressed by not being able to get through the locked door to go home and see mother, our aim is to soothe and relax. But sometimes the task is far from clear, and the case of Elsa (Box 6.2) is a good example. We generally worked on the premise that Elsa responded positively to arousal; she does after all spend the greater part of her waking day virtually comatose, and she does appear to enjoy her interludes of human interaction. But on this occasion we missed the mark, and the result was considerable over-arousal as far as we could tell. The dilemma in part is about finding a balance; finding a balance on each occasion of intervention, for the pivot point is always likely to be in a different place as moods and mental states wax and wane.

But there is another problem, and this is our major concern in this section. There is for some people in latter stage dementia, an intractable type of agitation which appears not to respond to intervention (see, for example, Boxes 6.3 and 6.4).

Violet's movement pattern seems to be a seated version of Maria's, with the exception of her gaze. Violet is able to sustain long, deep eye contact, and, perhaps for this reason, one feels that at least some level of communion

---

Box 6.3

Very occasionally Maria will sit quietly in a chair, but, for by far the greater part of each day, she is pacing the unit in considerable agitation. She walks with an unsteady gait, and always with a slight list to the left, which effectively means that she tends to walk around in circles. This pacing (or perhaps shuffling is a better word) is accompanied constantly by an agitated, breathy respiration, a puffing through cheeks and lips and an occasional grunt or whimper. Maria does not speak. When she meets furniture in her path, she will move slowly round it, picking up and wringing this plant or that ornament in a vacant fashion, and letting them tip over or fall to the floor. It is sometimes possible to engage eye contact, but this is random and fleeting, and Maria's gaze is generally fixed six inches above one's head. The presence and/or physical contact of a friend, relative or carer does not seem to impinge in any way upon this fixed cycle of agitated restlessness. No therapy has yet been found which has been able to make the slightest of dents in the impenetrable wall of this bubble.

Box 6.4

Violet seems to be afflicted with a similar problem to that of Maria, though she is chair-bound and unable to walk. She too is without language or speech, and spends much of her day moving constantly in her recliner chair. Her whole body makes infinitesimal movements, but there is a gross repetitive movement of her right leg in which the knee is raised and lowered, raised and lowered, brushing the other leg slightly in the process. There is a breathy, vocal accompaniment to this which can only be described as 'fuffing'.

is possible. Maria has been described as the most difficult client on the unit – difficult insofar as staff simply do not know how to try and relieve her agitation. It distresses everybody, and leaves an overwhelming sense of powerlessness and failure in its wake.

Agitated behaviours (or perhaps we can very reasonably refer to them as over-arousal) are a major problem in dementia care settings, and occur for a multiplicity of reasons. But perhaps we are wrong to describe the type of behaviour patterns exhibited by Maria and Violet (and many others in late dementia) as agitation. They certainly look like agitation. But maybe they are more correctly defined as movement disorders, or dyskinesias of neurological origin.

Paulson (1968), Brandon et al (1971) and Delwaide & Desseilles (1977) have all noted the prevalence of spontaneous dyskinesia in people who have dementia. Paulson has described postural changes, restless movements of hands and feet, respiratory tics, rocking, grimacing and mouth movements. These are very different from the comprehensive catalogue of 'agitations' described in Cohen-Mansfield's seminal work on the subject (1986, 1996), all of which are concerned with intentionality (or lack of it). It is important that we recognise the difference between the two for the sake of the focus of our treatment. Resolution is a realistic treatment aim for agitated behaviour, and seeks relaxation through occupational intervention. But if the problem is a dyskinesia of neurological origin – Kiernan (1987) suggests disruption within the basal ganglia – remission is extremely unlikely, and we need to appreciate this. If we take the dyskinesia of Parkinsonism as an example of an associated syndrome, we perhaps understand that we can do little more than attend as far as we are able to the person's physical comfort and psychological wellbeing. Paulson has observed that complex dyskinesias rarely disturb the person concerned, despite their unpleasant appearance. Nevertheless, whilst it is true that there is rarely evidence of pain, or of outward fatigue, most people in late dementia are no longer able to say how they feel, and until we know otherwise we should perhaps err on the side of assuming that this is a syndrome which, if it does not actually increase ill-being, does nothing to enhance wellbeing.

ORDER AND DISORDER?

What should be our response to the disorder of dementia?

The colleague with whom I had been dementia care mapping the unit described in Box 6.5 made no bones, later that day, about expressing her disgust. She was absolutely incensed at how staff had handled (or not handled) this mealtime, perceiving it as a total affront to the dignity of the residents. It was partly the physical mess, partly the noise and partly the general sense of chaos and disorder that she found so upsetting. What are the rights and wrongs here? This is a vexed issue for many dementia care workers. The superficial view would perhaps go along these lines: 'I always insisted that we sat down to the table as a family at mealtimes. I was brought up to have manners at the meal table and I brought my children up the same. When I am in a home, I hope people will care enough to remember that and help me keep my dignity'. We have probably all felt like this at one time or another. Who amongst us has never said, 'I hope I never get like that' or 'How could they ever let her get like that?'

This area of order and disorder in dementia must surely be one of the most difficult for carers to deal with, and offers a significant challenge to those who glibly idealise the person-centred approach. It is a fact of life that we are creatures of habit and routine, most of us entrenched in life-long patterns of activity from young adulthood onward, and unless there is considerable intrinsic motivation or external environmental pressure, we do not alter these patterns much over the life course.

There is no question that dementia incurs *dis*order; above everything it disrupts, upsets and overturns all those long-established modes of being and doing, for sufferer and for carer alike. We have in previous chapters described a person-centred approach which requires the carer to enter the 'other world' of the person with dementia; but in order to do that, the carer must not only have some understanding of the 'new order' of the dementing person, but also be able to accommodate to that with all its attendant disruption to the carer's own order and form. In practice, what this means is that what may appear to us as random and chaotic, may not be for the person with dementia, who may have found a new form and a different order in the context of his or her diminishing abilities.

Box 6.5

Lunch-time on the unit was formally over, but several residents were still seated at the table. Arthur had finished his meal and his plate had been removed; he kept trying to stand but appeared to have neither the strength nor the ability. Beatrice was finishing her drink from a feeder cup. Ernest, whose pudding plate had long since disappeared, was still eating imaginary plum crumble from the table with his spoon, with every appearance of enjoying it. Sylvia's plum crumble was half-eaten in the plate; she seemed to have forgotten it and was looking down at the side of her chair, fingering her skirt. There seemed to be food everywhere, on hands, around mouths, down bibs, in laps, smeared over tables, splodged on the floor. Chaos reigned, it seemed.

The chaotic scenario described in Box 4.1 left *me* feeling disturbed, disempowered and upset, but I cannot assume that the participants of that scene were experiencing a like feeling. The same might be said of my colleague in regard to the scenario in Box 6.5. Can we assume that because a person has custard on their cardigan, jam on their fingers and a tea puddle on the table, they are demeaned or diminished or reduced in self-esteem? The fact that we find this picture distasteful does not mean that they do; the fact that they themselves would once have found this picture distasteful, does not necessarily mean that they do now. This is where our 'person-centredness' is really laid on the line. Are we able to set aside our own distaste/disgust at this habit or that action, if it seems to be in some way valuable or important to the other? That should be our measure – the wellbeing of the individual, not levels of noise or mess or chaos.

This all seems at heart to be a matter of occupational identity (Perrin 1997b), that unique mix of occupations which personifies the individual at any given time in their lives. It is also a matter of our ability to perceive and understand and accept the changes to valued activities wrought by dementia. Beatrice, described in Box 6.5, was 'a lady'. She had been the wife of a diplomat; she entertained regularly in her younger years, and one assumes that it would have been silver service. Beatrice would have known the correct fold to a napkin, which fork to start with, how to crook the little finger. There is no comparison between the Beatrice of today and the Beatrice of 40 years ago – except perhaps in a fierce but silent independence. Today's Beatrice uses neither napkin nor fork, and rejects proffered cutlery. Nor will she be fed by another from a spoon, vigorously slapping aside any helping hand. All is partaken with fingers, squidged, mashed and liberally spread about, and a main meal invariably takes well over an hour. Is Beatrice demeaned; is she no longer a lady? We don't think so. The essence of Beatrice, an indomitable spirit, remains; it is her occupational identity that has changed. She still has the ability to will and to choose, and in her deepening dementia she clearly chooses, and at some level values, eating in this fashion. Beatrice would have been the first to say (40 years ago), 'Don't ever let me get like that'. But that was 40 years ago, and Beatrice has moved on. She is in essence still the same; the things she does are different.

We must as carers beware of imposing our order, our need for order, upon the person with dementia. We have spoken much of the return to childhood patterns in dementia; if we can give an assent to such an analogy, we might watch the toddler in the high chair feeding himself Marmite soldiers, and understand.

FAMILIARITY OR NOVELTY?

Which do we emphasise in our selection of activities?

We introduced in the last section a concept of occupational identity, for we believe that such a concept is fundamental to the provision of truly person-centred care. In dementia care generally, current health and social care screening prioritises the assessment of physical condition, family and social circumstances, environment, and mental and emotional integrity.

Considerably less attention is paid to the matter of occupational identity. This has thankfully begun to change in recent years, though we have to acknowledge that, even today, a few dotted lines on a form on which to indicate 'previous occupation' and 'hobbies and interests' is often the sum total of occupational information sought at assessment. For many elderly mentally impaired people who are already in institutional care, not even these meagre facts are known. But the tide is turning, and many centres now emphasise the need for a full occupational and social biography as an integral part of individual care planning. This is as it should be, for as we noted above, a person's occupational identity at any given time in their life is likely to determine those occupations in which they prefer to engage.

There is no question that for every one of our clients, we should be trying to build as full an occupational biography as possible. But we would want to include a note of caution here, for the tide which has swept in such an emphasis and interest in exploring the past, in reminiscence and life history and life story books, also has the potential to drown the importance of the present. Emphasis on the past can obscure the person of the here and now. Our client may have the same likes and dislikes as 10 or 20 or 30 years ago, but may well not – and we must be open to this. We cannot assume that because Anne liked to dance then, she does now; that because she always did the daily paper crossword, she will now; that because she was a great pastry-cook, she still has something invested in the kitchen today. Dementia changes a person's occupational identity, and we have a responsibility to our clients to ensure that we are as aware of what that identity is today, as we are of what it was yesterday. Of course, we have a responsibility to compile a biography, to enquire of friends, relatives and carers. But we have an equal responsibility to develop and maintain a current profile, and it may well be that friends and family are quite unable to assist us with this.

The key, as always, is finding a balance: bearing in mind what was, whilst remaining open to what is. We should not therefore feel that we must confine ourselves in therapeutic activity to those things which have been familiar to a person. We must be prepared to take the risk of exploring the novel and the unfamiliar. Not many of us cuddle dolls in the maturity of adulthood; a surprising number of people with dementia do. I well remember the discomfort of first taking a doll on to a residential unit. One lady who rarely put more than two words together looked at me in disgust exclaiming, 'Oh no, not a doll!'. Another lady took it wordlessly in her arms, held it tightly and fell asleep embracing it. If I hadn't taken the risk with the unfamiliar, one of those ladies would have missed a rare opportunity of warmth and attachment. Was she a 'doll person' in the past, as some of us are with teddy bears and soft toys? I don't know – but she is now. I remember too the lady with whom I tried all kinds of 'age appropriate' activities; she sat mute and depressed through them all. The day I brought a big beach ball on to the unit was the first I had ever seen her smile. She was transformed. I didn't know this lady well, but something about her told me she wasn't a champion beach ball player in early life. She is now.

The dementia that is inexorably changing every other aspect of a person's life, is changing occupational identity too. It is an insidious, slowly moving thing, and our task is to stay with it, constantly appraising and reappraising. Only in such a way can we be effective practitioners.

There is an additional principle of good occupational practice, which we have so far only touched on indirectly. Yet it is of such importance, that a book on occupational interventions in dementia would be incomplete without it. Chapter 7 looks at the place of non-verbal communication in dementia, and how the success or failure of a therapeutic intervention can often hinge upon the therapist's understanding and use of non-verbal mechanisms of communicating.

Key Points

- The process of carrying out an activity is set in the here and now; the product of an activity belongs to the future. In dementia, it is likely that 'here and now' experience is of more therapeutic value than future outcome.
- Activities set in a cognitive framework can be counterproductive as a dementia takes hold, and should be used with sensitivity and caution.
- Restlessness and agitation are a feature of dementia for many; the therapist must decide whether the agitation is a symptom of distress or of a dyskinesia of neurological origin, and direct intervention accordingly.
- The disorder and chaos of dementia is a challenge to the person-centred approach. Every carer must endeavour to understand noise and muddle and mess from the standpoint of the person with dementia.
- The concept of occupational identity is central to planning occupational intervention. The carer needs to recognise that occupational identity may change over the course of dementia.

References

Bexton W, Heron W, Scott T 1954 Effects of decreased variation in the sensory environment. Canadian Journal of Psychology 8(2):70–76

Birchmore T, Clague S 1983 A behavioural approach to reduce shouting. Nursing Times (April 20th):37–39

Bower H 1967 Sensory stimulation and the treatment of senile dementia. Medical Journal of Australia 1(22):1113–1119

Brandon S, McClelland H, Protheroe C 1971 A study of facial dyskinesia in a mental hospital population. British Journal of Psychiatry 118:171–184

Cleary A, Clamon C, Price M, Shullaw G 1988 A reduced stimulation unit: effects on patients with Alzheimer's disease and related disorders. The Gerontologist 28(4):511–514

Cohen-Mansfield J 1986 Agitated behaviors in the elderly: II, Preliminary results in the cognitively deteriorated. Journal of the American Geriatric Society 34(10):722–727

Cohen-Mansfield J 1996 Conceptualization of agitation: results based on the Cohen-Mansfield Agitation Inventory and the Agitation Behavior Mapping Instrument. International Psychogeriatrics 8(3):309–315

Delwaide P, Desseilles M 1977 Spontaneous buccolingual facial dyskinesia in the elderly. Acta Neurologica Scandinavica 56:256–262

Diamond M 1976 Anatomical brain changes produced by environment. In: McGaugh J, Petrinovich L (eds) Knowing, thinking and believing. Plenum Press, New York

Diamond M 1978 The aging brain: some enlightening and optimistic results. American Scientist 66:66–71

Greene J, Nichol R, Jamieson H 1979 Reality orientation with psychogeriatric patients. Behaviour Research and Therapy 17:615–617

Greene J, Timbury G, Smith R, Gardiner M 1983 Reality orientation with elderly patients in the community: an empirical evaluation. Age and Ageing 12:36–43

Hall G 1994 Caring for people with Alzheimer's disease using the conceptual model of progressively lowered stress threshold in the clinical setting. Nursing Clinics of North America 29(1):129–141

Hanley I, McGuire R, Boyd W 1981 Reality orientation and dementia: a controlled trial of two approaches. British Journal of Psychiatry 138:10–14

Kiernan J 1987 Introduction to neuroscience. J B Lippincott, Philadelphia

Ostwald M 1962 Nichomachean ethics. Bobbs-Merrill, New York

Paire J, Karney R 1984 The effectiveness of sensory stimulation for geropsychiatric inpatients. American Journal of Occupational Therapy 38(8):505–509

Paulson G 1968 'Permanent' or complex dyskinesias in the aged. Geriatrics 23:105–111

Perrin T 1997a The role and value of occupation in severe dementia. Unpublished PhD thesis, University of Bradford

Perrin T 1997b Occupational need in dementia care: a literature review and implications for practice. Health Care in Later Life 2(3):166–176

Rogers J, Marcus C, Snow T 1987 Maude: a case of sensory deprivation. American Journal of Occupational Therapy 41(10):673–676

Chapter 7

Non-verbal communication: the currency of wellbeing

INTRODUCTION

Non-verbal communication is one of those things which is so implicitly understood by every single one of us, almost from birth onwards, that we rarely give it a thought. Throughout life we abide slavishly by the cultural rules and conventions which we imbibe along with our mother's milk, and we are not usually awakened to its structures and mechanisms until we are presented with a communication problem – our own or that of another. By way of illustration, we might think of the child, who has learned to speak and use a conventional language generally by the age of 3 years. The language has in a sense grown with him; he has had no lessons, been taught no rules, he knows nothing of grammar and syntax. He communicates ably without even thinking about it. But ask him how he arrived at that place of competent communication; ask him to describe the mechanisms with which he imparts information satisfactorily to another or receives information from another; ask him to teach his skills to a person less able, and he won't have a clue. This is how most of us are with the matter of non-verbal language, well into adult life. But give us a communication problem of some sort, and we are forced into a position where we must acknowledge its existence and learn its workings. Dementia gives us just such a problem.

We know only too well that the advance of a dementia inexorably disrupts and may destroy verbal language and speech over the course of time. But we live in a culture and a time in which articulate facility with the written and spoken word is highly prized. Take that away from us, and most of us are like a fish out of water – removed from that natural and familiar environment in which we can live and move freely. Most of us, dare we acknowledge it, are afraid, at least initially, when we are first confronted by someone who can no longer respond to our verbal overtures in ways we have come to expect from past experience. If we are not afraid, we are at least discomfited, for such a situation diminishes our competence, renders us vulnerable, threatens our control, and, perhaps most worrying of all, has a powerful potential to make us look a fool. We have all been there. It usually happens when there is an audience – of our colleagues, our friends or uncomprehending passers-by. The person with dementia confronts us, full of emotion and intent, with a stream of jumbled incoherence to which we are clearly expected to make a response. What kind of response do we give which will satisfy the challenger, extricate ourselves from the situation, and save face at the same time? We are only too uncomfortably aware that conventional language is usually redundant at such a time, but this is precisely where our supplementary, non-verbal mechanisms of communication come into their own. If we have not recognised them before, we need to recognise them now; if we have not learned their concepts and constructs before, we need to learn them now. This is all we have left, and if we do not assimilate the subtleties and intricacies of this language, we might as well forget about planned therapeutic interventions. For this is the currency with which we trade, and nobody is going to 'buy' our therapeutic interventions unless they are presented in a language which is understood.

Non-verbal communication is perhaps best understood as operating in an interplay of culture, environment and person. We might think of it as in Figure 7.1. It is commonly assumed that human beings are the sole transmitters of information and messages, and without doubt we have an immense potential in this area.

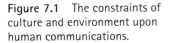

Figure 7.1 The constraints of culture and environment upon human communications.

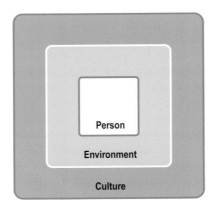

'There seems to be no agent more effective than another person in bring-ing the world for oneself alive, or, by a glance, a gesture, or a remark, shrivelling up the reality in which one is lodged.' (Goffman 1961)

However, messages are also powerfully carried by the environment and the culture around us.

'The physical environment unremittingly offers us possibilities of experi-ence, or curtails them. The fundamental human significance of archi-tecture stems from this. The glory of Athens … and the horror of so many features of the modern megalopolis is that the former enhances and the latter constricts man's consciousness.' (Laing 1967)

Imagine then the impact of some long-stay environments on the con-sciousness and wellbeing of people who have dementia; people who, argu-ably, are more tuned in to non-verbal messages than verbal.

What is the message being conveyed by the environment described in Box 7.1? Well, surely something like – 'You are not worth much. You will die soon anyway. The sooner the better'. Clearly, it does not need a person to come and say to the inhabitants of that ward – 'You are not worth visiting/spend-ing money on/being clean for.' The physical environment says it all. And the message of the physical environment is supported in turn by a message from the prevailing socioeconomic culture which has determined that the ward will close. And *this* message says that we must move with the times, live more cost-effectively, save money – buildings and services take priority over people.

Nevertheless we must not lose sight of the fact that it is people who shape both environment and culture; environment and culture can only pass on the message that we as individuals or as a society permit. The person is at the core.

So how are messages reciprocated in a non-verbal manner? How does it all work? How can we ensure that channels of communion between ourselves and the people with whom we work are, and remain, open and uncluttered?

The greater part of this chapter is concerned with an exploration of the way we use and interpret body and voice, but effective communications are not just reliant upon a knowledge and use of this or that movement

---

Box 7.1

On the ward that I work on now, there is a huge black unspoken 'non-verbal' looming above us all. The ward is closing; it will not be replaced; the beds will be absorbed by two other wards on the opposite side of town. The ward is scruffy and smelly. Paint is flaking off the ceiling. The silk flowers have stood on the windowsill for so long they have been bleached a dirty yellow by the sun. The tear in the curtain has never been mended. Relatives' visits are rare; consultant visits rarer. The incidence of falls has gone up, which is strange because there is a pall of lethargy over the place which makes you feel as though nothing ever happens here. Actually, not much does beyond the conventional routine of nursing care.

or gesture or voice tone. These are important – hence we will concentrate upon them. But we must first say that the essence, the essential element of effective communications is actually a matter of integrity – what we **believe** must match what we **say** (verbally) which must match what we **do** with our body and voice. Any discrepancy will engender a mixed message, and mixed messages serve only to confuse and threaten. Mixed messages are clogged channels. I have a poignant cartoon which I cut out of a social work journal several years ago. Two elderly ladies are sitting together in a living room chatting over a cup of tea. One is saying to the other, 'My social worker is very interested in gardening – she always looks out of the window when I'm talking to her'. This is not integrity – it is dishonesty. It is a mismatch of what the social worker believes, says and does. And we who look upon this scene know that the elderly lady also knows that – maybe only at a subliminal level, but she knows it. The message she has received is, 'Your garden is more important to me than you are'. Or possibly even, 'You are of so little value to me that I would rather look at anything but you'. Powerful messages – which close down the channels of communion.

Look again at the illustration of Julie and Audrey in Box 4.4 – not a dissimilar scenario to the cartoon described above. Communion was established first and foremost because Julie really liked Audrey, because she believed that Audrey was a fellow human being worthy of attention and consideration, and because what she did matched what she felt.

In the case described in Box 7.2, neither Amy nor I ever had to put any of our initial antipathy into words, but we both knew exactly how the

Box 7.2	
	When I first came to work on Ward 10, the biggest problem I had was a lady called Amy. Amy was very confident, upper class, verbose. She always seemed to have the upper hand with me and she frightened me. I got on her nerves with my polite 'therapist' approach, and I'm pretty sure she viewed me as a female rival in the group; she held power in the ward society, and so did I, though of a quite different nature. Often she would call me a hussy or such like, and responded to all my endeavours in a resistive fashion. If asked to join in, she'd opt out; if asked to opt out she'd join in. It was difficult for me to express my anger, frustration and irritation with her, or the sense of failure she provoked in me. Therapists aren't allowed to give vent to these feelings, and so we got off to a bad start because I couldn't be authentic and honest with her. She knew this and mistrusted me. Ultimately, it was a soft cuddly toy that came to our rescue – two in fact. Amy had a long-standing relationship with two big white fluffy cats – her 'boys' she called them; and they went everywhere with her, one under each arm. Often, they were my only real point of contact with her; I made as much of them as I could, and they gradually came to act as a bridge between us. Slowly, she came to trust my regard for them, and appreciate my capacity to enjoy them with her. The day she asked me to look after them for a few minutes was a big day for me; it meant we had truly achieved an authentic relationship of mutual regard.

other felt. We knew it because of that mismatch of inner attitudes, word and actions; and that mismatch effectively blocked the channels of any real communion between us for some considerable time.

What of the person with dementia? Does cognitive incapacity impinge upon a person's ability to understand and use non-verbal means of communication? It seems not. It seems that as far as we can tell, a person with dementia is just as able (if not more so) to understand and assimilate non-verbal communications as an unimpaired person. In a piece of empirical research that must surely be ahead of its time, Hoffman et al (1985) demonstrated that:

- non-verbal communication abilities of people with dementia are comparable to those of unimpaired people
- even people with severe dementia are responsive to emotional undertones in the environment
- positive affective non-verbal messages elicit positive verbal and non-verbal responses in people with dementia
- negative affective non-verbal messages elicit withdrawal and apparent discomfort
- social conventions are apparent even in people with severe dementia.

Hoffman et al conclude that 'even persons who have completely lost language capabilities are still as responsive to non-verbal communications as the non-demented'. They also go as far as to suggest that the cognitive losses of dementia may actually serve to sharpen non-verbal communication abilities, rather as a loss of visual acuity sharpens the remaining senses to a keener sensitivity. A more recent study (Hubbard et al 2002) supports Hoffman's findings.

These are critically important observations, which leave us with no excuses for not becoming diligent students of this supplementary language. They offer a challenge to the careless practice of those who attribute little or no understanding to people with dementia, and a powerful incentive to make the best possible use of that which remains.

So where do we start? Let's go back to our first analogy of the child *imbibing* his first knowledge of the language. He may of course never get beyond that, nor wish to do so. He may speak the language perfectly well, and yet never learn how to spell, or recognise the different parts of speech, or know how to parse sentences. But if he should be going on in later life to become a linguist or an author or a teacher, he will certainly need to acquire a deeper understanding of the structure of language; indeed he will probably be well motivated to dig deeper. The starting point for this child is usually a book of English usage and a good teacher. And here our analogy falls down rather, for our non-verbal language is not taught in school in the conventional manner of other languages; it is not on the national curriculum; you can't take an A-Level in it.

Nevertheless, much is known and has been discovered about non-verbal communication over the years, and we are about to turn our attention to this. But the key to learning any language is something we don't have to go searching the schools and bookshops for; the key is in listening to others, listening and establishing individual and cultural patterns in what we hear. It is also in listening to ourselves and shaping our own communications to match those we are receiving from the other person. With verbal language we listen; with non-verbal language we watch; there isn't a great deal of difference, it's a tuning in. What we are saying here really is that the art of learning the language of non-verbal communication, is in becoming a skilled observer of others, and an honest critic of ourselves. Two questions must always be at the forefront of our minds in dementia care: what message is this person trying to deliver to me, and what message am I giving (or trying to give) to this person?

What we attempt to deal with in this chapter, is to highlight those non-verbal mechanisms with which we all communicate information, and to draw attention to their use and misuse in dementia care. Non-verbal mechanisms of communication rely on the use of body and voice. We will deal with the body first.

HOW DO WE USE OUR BODY IN ITS RELATIONSHIP OR PROXIMITY TO ANOTHER PERSON (OR PERSONS)?

It is well known that each of us carries around about us a set of invisible social barriers, rather like a series of concentric circles, which determine who gets close to us and who doesn't. The actual permitted distances vary from culture to culture, but in western society generally, we tend to deal in fairly extended distances. In professional/client contact, we need to keep anything from four to twelve feet between us for comfort. In informal interactions between friends, this distance is something between eighteen inches and four feet; and only intimates are permitted within the eighteen inch circumference (Hall 1966). The inappropriate person who invades those set barriers causes us grave discomfort, for what they have done is to violate a socially acceptable norm. Our response is immediate withdrawal. I once found myself backed right across my kitchen and up against the sink unit by a boiler repair man who was consistently invading my own personal 18 inches of intimate space. Not only was I in considerable discomfort, but I was also very confused. My first thought, that this might be a sexual overture, I discarded; for even when drawn to full height he was still a foot shorter than I and his verbal communications were in no way sexually loaded. Ultimately (when I had extricated myself) I concluded that either he had never learned social graces, or he had been brought up in a different cultural setting. But the clear mismatch between what he was saying (entirely acceptable) and what he was doing (entirely unacceptable) was very confusing, and I never did decide what the message was that I was supposed to have received.

The situation described in Box 7.3 was, I believe, an issue of Keith's personal space and my invasion of it. Keith and I have a good relationship; most of the time I would describe it as a relationship between friends which, according to the research indicated above, would allow a comfortable distance of between two and four feet. This does indeed describe how we normally behave with each other. As his carer though, I sometimes

Box 7.3

Keith and I had gone down to the Leisure Centre to play squash. We had been playing energetically for 20 minutes or so when suddenly Keith came over faint and wobbly. I thought he was going to fall and managed to get him safely to the floor. I wasn't sure what this was but after a short while he seemed recovered, though he was confused and embarrassed and shrugged off an offer of help from one of the attendants. It was a short walk to the nearest chair in the coffee bar, and as he was swaying and still wobbly I felt I needed to hang on to him in case he should stumble or fall. So I did the thing that felt most natural for me and which I thought would draw the least attention – I held his hand. Unusually in such circumstances there was no responding pressure – it was like holding a dead hand. And the hand was rapidly withdrawn just as soon as a chair was safely in sight. I realised that with the best of intentions I had overstepped the mark and invaded Keith's sense of personal space.

have to invade that 18 inches of intimate space, for example, at home when he needs assistance with dressing. On these occasions he tolerates such invasions usually with equanimity, intuitively understanding that in such situations the conventional rules are suspended. This time I was again attempting to respond as carer, but the circumstances were different. I had again invaded intimate space, but this time the action was unsolicited, in a public place where people might be looking, and at a time when he was clearly feeling more vulnerable than usual. It caused him immediate and obvious discomfort, and caused me to think again. As soon as I restored the distance balance to the three or four feet afforded by the coffee table, it gave him the (literal) space he needed re-assert normal proceedings.

This was a small thing which appeared readily forgotten and made no lasting impact on our relationship. But it was reminder of how subtle and how powerful are the unwritten rules which govern interactions, and how sensitive we need to be when people no longer have the conventional verbal language to deal with the messages we convey with our bodies.

HOW DO WE USE PHYSICAL CONTACT IN OUR COMMUNICATIONS WITH ANOTHER PERSON?

Physical contact is, in a way, an extension of all that we have written about above in the context of bodily proximity. Physical contact also has its own set of culturally determined rules: who may touch whom, when, and how, and where. There are circumstances, in health care settings for example, where touch may be devoid of emotion and coldly clinical. But generally speaking, touch is always about strong emotion, both positive and negative. It has the power to convey strong emotion, and it has the power to engender strong emotion. I would have forgotten all about my remark to Betty (Box 7.4) that day, if I had not seen her reciprocate the compliment,

Box 7.4

> There was something different about Betty today. She was wearing a beautiful white lacy cardigan – clean and fresh. She looked really lovely. So I took her hand and told her so. 'Do I? Oh, thank you', she said and smiled. Just a few minutes later, I happened to notice her pass Molly in the corridor. She paused in front of Molly, stroked her cheek softly and lovingly, and said, 'You look lovely'. Molly too smiled, glowed rather gently, and moved on.

and the feeling, towards Molly. It was as though love was being passed on through a touch of the hand. But other feelings are passed on through touch too (Box 7.5).

Though there is no pun intended, we have to say that touch can be difficult to handle. Its emotional loading means that we need to have a clear understanding of the cultural rules, and an acute sensitivity to what touch means to every individual. This is a matter requiring increasing sensitivity as a dementia advances, not just because of the growing number of physical care tasks which we need to administer, but also because of the return to childhood needs, to which we have alluded much in previous chapters. As a person moves through the latter stages of a dementia, there is an increasing need for holding, massaging, caressing and stroking. This is what a mother does with her child. But here there is an intimacy of family relationship that nobody would question. Those of us in care settings are

Box 7.5

> Doug had always been affectionate with staff, but since his wife died five months previously, this had started to get out of hand. Gestures which at one time had been understood, and managed, by staff as a fatherly warmth or perhaps a harmless flirtation, were increasingly permeated with sexual overtones. It had come to a point where the physical or nursing care that Doug required could not be carried out by female staff without a hand going up the skirt or down the blouse. Where possible, Doug was attended by one of the two male care staff, but inevitably there were many occasions when this was just not possible. Some of the women on the staff dealt with this better than others. Some were repelled and disgusted, and resorted to avoidance or verbal abuse. Others understood that Doug was lonely, missing his wife terribly, and becoming increasingly sexually frustrated. But understanding that didn't necessarily make the situation any easier to handle. Doug's demands were unpleasant and unacceptable, and he was effectively alienating himself from everybody. Those staff who really did care for him, and felt deeply for his needs, were faced with an insoluble dilemma – a man whose deepest needs were for warmth, affection and love, but whose expression of those needs exiled the only people who could in some measure meet them.

not family, and we need to exercise caution. We live in a rather litigious age in which there are risks for adults in their expressions of intimacy and physical contact, since these can be misconstrued as inappropriately sexual in orientation. Those of us who are providers of intimate physical care need to be alert to the potential for difficulties in this area.

WHAT IMPORTANCE DO WE ATTACH TO EYE CONTACT IN OUR INTERACTIONS?

Eye contact has been well researched over the years, and seems to have two principal functions. It is strongly associated with liking, and it has been found (unsurprisingly) that we look much more at people we like than at people we dislike, and that we look longer at people we like more than at people we like less. It also has a role in regulating the flow of communication, signalling turn-taking between speaker and listener. Looking occurs more intensively in the listener than in the speaker, and acts as a social reinforcer, assuring people of our attention.

We felt that Maria (Box 7.6) was saying to us very clearly that she liked this lady who was sitting with her and talking to her, that she liked her very

---

Box 7.6

It was PAT (Pets As Therapy) Dog visiting day, and Sally, the Cavalier King Charles spaniel, was doing her rounds. Most of the residents of the ward were responding well, some with great warmth and affection, and we had assumed that Maria would too. Although Maria has an advanced dementia and no longer speaks, she does nevertheless retain an interest in people and events, and is well able to initiate contact with others; we thought she would love the dog. Sally was placed gently in her lap, snuffled and shuffled about a bit to make herself comfortable, and nuzzled Maria's hand wanting a bit of attention. But Maria could not give that attention, for she appeared to be quite unable to perceive or appreciate the animal. Sally's owner Janet sat at the side of Maria's chair for ten or fifteen minutes, vainly trying to draw Maria's attention to the dog. She even moved the dog bodily at one point to try and bring it within Maria's line of vision, but to no avail. Maria seemed to be totally oblivious to Sally's presence, despite the fact that she must surely have felt the weight of the dog on her lap, and one hand was actually holding the dog's leg. It seemed to those of us who observed, that the reason Maria could not engage with the dog at all, was because she was too much engaged with Janet. For the whole of the period that Sally and Janet were with her, her gaze was what can only be described as 'locked' into Janet's, and would not be diverted to anything else. Wherever Janet moved, Maria's eyes remained on hers. There was no particular accompanying facial expression, except once or twice a brief smile. But the intensity, and, one felt, intimacy, of that gaze was to the exclusion of all else. It didn't matter that there was a warm, cuddly, wriggly thing clamouring for her attention right under her nose; Maria had made human contact, achieved communion, and in her world right now, nothing else mattered.

much, and was truly appreciative of the attention Janet was giving her. In her turn, she was repaying Janet with her full concentration, not because what was being said was making any sense to her necessarily, but because there was a very mutual pleasure in togetherness. We need to be able to use eye contact. The eye has been called the window of the soul, and there is some substance to this metaphor. When all other avenues of communion are gone, eye contact often remains, and while this is the case, it somehow feels possible to retain a thread of contact. When it is gone, it is rather as though the person inside the body has gone over the edge to be seen no longer. Establishing eye contact is a vital prerequisite to any therapeutic intervention. We need to be saying clearly to people, 'I like you, and I'm listening to you'. And likewise we may be fairly sure that if we are not getting a reasonably substantial amount of gaze in return, we cannot be confident that they like *us* and are listening to *us*; we may not have established sufficient contact to be able to render our intervention therapeutic.

WHAT IMPORTANCE SHOULD WE ATTACH TO FACIAL EXPRESSION?

Facial expression is a library of emotions, but how often do we trouble to read the open books in front of us, and how much concern do we have about the messages we display on our own faces in the therapeutic situation? In Ben's case (Box 7.7), why had nobody looked at his face, and troubled themselves to identify and understand the distress that it showed? Why had staff jumped immediately to the conclusion that this was the dementia speaking? Probably because they had not fully understood the role of facial expression in non-verbal communications, and probably

Box 7.7

Ben was a genial man with a sunny disposition. He no longer had any useful language left, but this didn't seem to trouble him; he always had a ready smile for everyone who passed his way. He was well-liked by staff, who often sought him out to spend time with him. But he seemed to be turning aggressive of late. Nobody could pinpoint the time of the change, but it had seemed to happen fairly suddenly. He looked miserable these days, and sat slumped in his chair most of the time. He avoided eye contact, and it was hard to get a word out of him. He had started to lash out at staff, for no apparent reason, although it seemed to be mostly in situations where they were offering some physical care. There was a general agreement that his dementia had taken a sudden downturn; he had been on the unit a long time and maybe it was to be expected. He was starting to earn description as an aggressive man, and new agency staff on the unit were warned to be on their guard. This situation looked set to continue, until the return of a charge nurse who had been away on training for some while. He was so shocked at the change in Ben that he ordered an immediate health screening. It was found that Ben had been walking around on a fractured femur for the last three weeks.

because blaming dementia for all the quirky things that happen to people means that we don't have to exert ourselves to look for other reasons.

Facial expression has also been well researched in recent years, and the work of Ekman et al (Ekman & Friesen 1969, Ekman et al 1983) stands out as having particular significance. Facial expression is our prime means of expressing emotion; Ekman et al have demonstrated that there are at least seven facial expressions of emotion which are universally recognised across cultures: the most common are happiness, sadness, surprise, fear, anger, disgust and interest. This is important information; it tells us that no matter what the nationality or culture of the person with whom we are communicating, each will recognise the other's basic facial expression. We have no excuse for not reading and at least in some measure understanding the emotions which are registering upon another's face. The first question the staff on the unit should have been asking themselves is, 'Last week Ben was happy (i.e. smiling, laughing, eye contact, face animated), this week Ben is miserable (i.e. mouth turned down, eyes lowered, face static) – what has made the difference?'. And perhaps the second question the team should have asked is, 'Are we delivering any particular messages to Ben through the expressions upon our own faces, to which he might be responding?'.

The strong association between emotion and facial expression also determines that facial expressions play a significant role in the forming and maintaining of relationships. We began to see this too in Ben's case; for relationships were beginning to sour, and he was beginning to experience rejection and ostracism, and dismissal as a nasty old man. And this had only taken three weeks.

There is, of course, no question that our acquisition of social conventions across the life span enables most of us to exert conscious control over those expressions which appear on our faces. Most of us, for example, would be able to modify the natural expressions of glee and elation we felt on passing an exam, if we know that the good friend we are with has failed that same exam. And who amongst us has not at one time or another put on a smiley, all's-well-with-the-world front (though we felt like death) because someone has arranged a birthday party for us, or because great-aunt Gladys is visiting from Australia. But these overlays are indeed fronts, or masks, and require a significant cognitive application to put them into effect. People with dementia do not have the cognitive ability to construct and wear such masks, and therefore to engage in such subtleties, and this actually makes our own job as carer that much easier. What you see is what you get.

HOW DO WE USE GESTURE IN THE COMMUNICATION OF INFORMATION?

Gesture is a very powerful means of delivering messages, and emphasising intention. There are essentially three types of gesture: the emblem, the illustrator and the reinforcer (Ekman & Friesen 1969). Emblems are bodily movements, such as a wave, or an element of sign language, which have a direct verbal equivalent. Illustrators emphasise the content of that which is spoken: for example, the finger pointing of the person giving directions, the pounding of the lectern by the political speaker, the miming of object shape/size, etc. when it is not present in the environment. Reinforcers are those head nods and hand movements which help regulate the flow of conversation.

The vigorous head-shake in the scenario described in Box 7.8 was an emblem, having a direct verbal equivalent, understood throughout the western world as a negative – 'No. Definitely not'. And the more vigour in the head-shake, the more emphatic the negative. It is unsurprising therefore that the message I received standing at the church doorway was, 'No. You can't come in'. And that message, uncontradicted by any verbal message in the first few seconds, was quite sufficient first to confuse me totally, and then to anger me considerably. Who did this woman think she was? Well, of course, that rapidly became clear, and the situation resolved, but just for a minute I was completely thrown. A small incident, but one which illustrated for me the power of gesture.

Box 7.8

A recent job change has meant that I have had to move during the last year from the north to the south of the country. This has meant not only having to find a new house, in which I could be as comfortable as the last, but having to find a new church as well, in which also I could be as comfortable as the last. To that end, I decided one Sunday evening to attend a service at a small church in the village to which we moved. Aiming for the usual 6.30 start, I arrived about 6.20, and judging by music coming from inside it sounded as though the service had already started. No matter, I thought, and tried the handle of the door. It wouldn't budge. I tried again, and must have been rattling rather loudly, for suddenly the door was opened from the inside to reveal a lady framed in the doorway. She looked at me. 'Can I come in?', I whispered, conscious that proceedings had already started within. She shook her head vigorously. I was stunned. I had never been refused entrance to a church service before; most churches are only too keen to welcome you in and pull you over the threshold. In the space of milliseconds, all manner of thoughts ran through my head. Didn't they allow anyone in after 6.15? Wasn't I wearing the right clothes? Did I need a password? Had I stumbled upon some kind of segregationist sect? Then the lady leant towards me. 'Are you coming to church?', she whispered. 'Hopefully', I whispered back. She stood back and let me through. It wasn't until I was safely seated in the back row of the stalls, that I had a chance to take another look at this lady. As I watched her out of the corner of my eye, opening the door for other late-comers, and later taking her own place a few rows further down, it gradually dawned on my consciousness that she was vigorously shaking her head at least once every couple of minutes. Actually, what she had was a very unfortunate nervous tic.

But what of the dementia care setting? How do we use gesture with our clients? Well, there are of course many universally understood gestures, such as the one above, and it is likely that our clients will retain an appreciation of these well into a dementia. We need to give thought to how we might mime certain objects and actions in situations where a person has lost the ability to appraise our verbal descriptions. It is a good discipline to get used to supplementing our verbal instructions with mime, for, as we have seen in earlier chapters, people with dementia retain the use of symbol long after more complex cognitive functions have gone, and the pictorial language of gesture is a useful adjunct to that which we convey verbally.

In addition, however, each of us as an individual has a range of gestures which are unique to ourselves. There will be similarities person to person, but nobody does it quite like us. Our first task is to learn the idiosyncrasies of gesture in our clients: what they do that is entirely their own, how they do it, when they do it, and under what circumstances. The second task is to learn our own. It is not, of course, always easy to know what those gestures are or how they appear to others, for we cannot see ourselves, and most of them are used subconsciously. But today with all our modern technology, we have no excuse for not knowing what we do. We have video. And in training colleges where people are going to be facing the public as a part of their job, video is in common use for this specific purpose – so that people should know just how they appear, and what messages they send, to others. We need to be using video in dementia care training and research.

OF WHAT RELEVANCE IS BODY POSTURE IN NON-VERBAL COMMUNICATIONS?

What does posture mean? Posture might perhaps be described as a 'whole body gesture'. As we use parts of our bodies to communicate information in certain ways, so we also use our whole body. Posture is the position of body and limbs, and associated muscle tone, understood as a whole. It is a symbol perhaps, of emotional state, and conveys certain attitudes.

Even without knowing Gwen and Edie (Box 7.9), most of us have sufficient understanding of postural indicators to make a good guess at their respective personalities and/or states of mind. Gwen is an anxious, rather nervous person, meticulous about cleanliness and hygiene and order, which tend to dominate her life. She has no confidence, rarely speaks unless spoken to, rarely moves unless invited. She is enclosed, buttoned up, afraid of the world. Edie doesn't care about anything very much. She is at ease with the world; does and says what she wants, when she wants, regardless of anybody else. She is the epitome of 'laid-back-ness'.

We need of course, to beware of reading too much into posture, but it is a useful starting point in our interactions. If Gwen appears muscularly tense and rigid, perhaps she is under stress; maybe we need to go carefully at our introduction, maybe we need to explore the stress. Edie is probably somebody we can be freer with. Her posture is relaxed and open; she is probably open to contact, maybe would relish a challenge. And as with

Box 7.9

Gwen and Edie usually sit in adjacent chairs. Gwen is in a smart tailored dress, belt neatly fastened, shoe laces carefully tied. She sits bolt upright, knees and feet together, leaning slightly forward. Hands are folded in the centre of her lap. Edie is in a rather crumpled pleated skirt and a baggy jumper with coffee stains down the front. She sprawls rather than sits; her bottom is on the front edge of the chair and she is half-sitting half-lying back into it. Legs are crossed, foot swinging, arms propped along the arm-rests. When Gwen gets up to walk about, it is in rigid, controlled movements, small, tight steps, hands either clasped in front of her or clutching her handbag tightly. When Edie gets up to walk about, she unfolds her legs, glides out of the chair and into a smooth easy stride. A graphic picture of contrasts.

Box 7.10

Richard hit a nurse yesterday. He stood up and hit her as she was trying to deal with Norma. In the hiatus that followed, what we failed to appreciate until much later was the posture of the nurse, and how that might have been perceived by Richard. Richard had been a prisoner of war, and his experience of authority figures is therefore probably quite different to ours. What he saw was a strong, large, powerful person towering over a vulnerable old lady. He had stepped in to rescue her, to defend her from being hurt by the authority figure.

gesture, we need to know what the messages are that we communicate to our clients, as well as they to us.

We should not forget that if posture gives us our first information about the person we are just about to talk to, so it gives them their first information about who we are too. We need not think that we are the only readers of body language (Box 7.10). It will be a mutual appraisal; intuitive on their part perhaps, rather than cognitive, but as accurate as ours nevertheless

WHAT IS CONVEYED THROUGH VOICE – ASIDE FROM WORDS?

Words must surely be the smallest part of what we say, for we can speak the same words over and over again, and make them mean something different on each occasion. Consider the following simple phrase, overheard in a department store – 'I love this jacket'. Depending on how the phrase is spoken, how the voice is used, it can mean any number of different things. Different words may be stressed:

- *I* love this jacket – i.e. I love this jacket – my friend here doesn't.
- I *love* this jacket – i.e. I really, really like this jacket.

- I love *this* jacket – i.e. I love this jacket – not that one.
- I love this *jacket* – i.e. I love the jacket – don't think much of the rest.
- *I love this jacket* (shouted really loudly) – i.e. Look what you've done to it – it's ruined!
- I love this jacket (spoken very softly) – i.e. I can't throw it away – it reminds me of how he used to be.

Words are dependent for their meaning on volume of voice, rate of speech, intonation, pitch – we need to listen as much for these voice qualities as for the words themselves. They can signal emotion, add emphasis and convey attitudes.

It didn't matter that Henry (Box 7.11) had only these few apparently random words. The meaning was absolutely clear from the volume and the staccato delivery. They were not spoken; they were indeed spat out, as one would rid oneself of a distasteful mouthful. The words were helpful; they gave us an idea of where to start exploring. But we didn't actually need them to be able to understand that Henry was in extremis – angry, frightened, rejected, humiliated. John (Box 7.12) had even fewer intelligible words than Henry, but they were quite superfluous anyway. The staff nurse was responding with 'mmmms' and 'uh-huhs' and 'reallys?', taking her lead from John's intonations, mirroring his emphases and emotions in her voice. When he was laughing, she would laugh; when he grew serious, so would she. And so the conversation went on, richly rewarding for John, which is what matters, if not for the staff nurse.

If we have never developed listening skills before, we need to in dementia. We do need to give attention to such words as there are (more of this

---

Box 7.11

Henry was angry. His wife had left him at the day hospital and he was furious. Henry wasn't able to speak properly, but he was able to spit out the words 'this camp' and 'how dare they' and other single, apparently inappropriate words. It turned out that Henry had been in a prison camp during the war. 'This camp' was no better than that; it symbolised all that he was afraid of.

Box 7.12

John had waylaid the staff nurse and was talking nineteen to the dozen – though nobody knew what about. Somebody listening who was unable to speak English, would have been absolutely clear that this was an intensely pleasurable and animated conversation between two articulate people, about something obviously of considerable importance to John. Actually, it was gobbledegook, a meaningless jumble of words and phrases – to us at any rate. Not to John. To John, there was no question that this conversation was full of purpose, full of meaning, full of pleasure.

below), but we need to learn to read sound. We need to learn to use it also. The words that John's staff nurse was using were actually of little import to John. As far as we could tell, he wasn't able to understand them sufficiently to embrace them in his responses. But she *was* using sound, and using it very effectively if John's responses were anything to go by. Her voice was undulating over the scale, questioning, affirming, teasing, confidential, as she matched John's own inflexion and intonation. It is eminently possible to have a sustained and richly rewarding conversation between two parties without a lucid word being spoken on either side. Such is the power of the voice.

OF WHAT SIGNIFICANCE IS METAPHOR IN COMMUNICATION?

The rest of this chapter deals with the use of metaphor in the communications of people with dementia. Metaphor is of course about words and meanings of words, and, as such, is probably a little out of place in a chapter on non-verbal communication. But it is important that we look at it, and this seems to be the best place to do so; for although metaphor uses words, it is not about words used in a conventional manner. It is about words used as images, to convey messages in symbolic fashion.

We believe that, in the case described in Box 7.13, Frank was using metaphor to make a statement to the world. Frank's dementia was such that he was not able to articulate his thoughts and feelings in a conventional manner. But we believe that despite his cognitive disability, he was still able to deal in pictures and images set in his brain from many years ago.

Box 7.13

The music was good, and two or three couples had come together and started to move around the day centre floor. I was watching Frank, who was standing aside from the rest of the group, staring out of the window. I went over, and asked him if he would like to dance. Frank has only a handful of stereotyped phrases left, and I was unsure what kind of a reply I would get. He turned towards me and there were tears in his eyes. I put my hand on his arm and asked if he was alright. He looked at me thoughtfully for a few seconds, then grabbed me in a dance hold and started to waltz me erratically around the room. As we danced he would sing loudly over and over again, 'I'm only a bird in a cage. I'm only a bird in a cage'. I puzzled greatly over this in the car on the way home. For the actual line of the song that he was singing is, of course, 'I'm only a bird in a gilded cage'. He was singing exactly the right tune for the words, except that he was omitting the two-syllable word gilded, and its associated two notes. Had he forgotten the correct line? I thought that was unlikely; one can understand that he may well have lost other lines in the song, but music and song is deeply embedded in long-term memory. Why should he lose one word of a line that he otherwise knew and sang perfectly? And why was this line sung so frequently, in such a repetitive manner?

We believe that what Frank was wanting to say to the world was, 'I am a bird. I can still fly, I can still sing. But I am imprisoned in a cage, and the cage is called dementia. There is nothing gilded about this cage'. That is our belief – subjective of course, for there is no way that we can prove that this is what Frank is wanting to say. But we believe this because we feel that very little of that which is said or done by a person with dementia is random; most of it has meaning if we can but explore and understand.

Metaphor provides us with another avenue for understanding the language of dementia. But it is dependent upon our investment of meaning in the speech and actions of the person with dementia (Box 7.14). It won't work if our belief about the topsy-turvy communications of dementia is that they are flawed, or random, or mad. If we can believe in meaning, we can believe in metaphor; and if we can believe in metaphor, we have another tool in the tool-kit.

A metaphor, strictly speaking, is a figure of speech in which a word or a phrase denoting one kind of object or idea is used in place of another to suggest a likeness. It is used in literature to illustrate or illumine, and it has a close association with parable and allegory, an illustrative story designed to convince the hearer of a certain idea or concept. It is in effect a teaching mechanism, whose object is to enlighten those who wish to understand. Perhaps this is how we might best understand metaphor in dementia care. Our person with dementia cannot tell us a story or elaborate a rationale. He uses what he has left to make us understand what it is he would say, if only he had the ability.

There is no question, of course, that some of the 'parables' we see worked out in the course of our everyday practice in dementia are very difficult to understand. Those with a brain that thinks logically, in straight lines, are often not the best people to interpret the parables. Those who

---

Box 7.14

Irene was a young woman with a dementia that had been triggered by a loss of oxygen to her brain during a hysterectomy operation. She lived in a loop of anxiety. She would sit on her chair, jump suddenly as though she had just remembered an awful thought, and rush to her room to be sick. A few moments later she would return to her chair for the entire pattern to start over again. Things improved over the year, as her tolerance for being in a group increased. With the increased tolerance came relationships with others, and she became the girlfriend of another resident who spoiled and cared for her. On a summer's day I walked through the park with her. We chatted about this and that, and then to my surprise she announced with real joy how thrilled she was that her mother had come back (mother was dead, in fact). In the 'old days' I might have reported this to the nursing team as some sign of psychosis or delusion, but I instinctively felt that I understood what she was saying. I checked out my hunch. 'Do you mean that you are feeling safe and loved now, and that you weren't before?' 'Yes', she replied, 'That's exactly it. You've got it.'

Box 7.15

Ronald was becoming a problem in group activities, and staff were beginning to feel that they would have to start excluding him from activities which involved food in any way. For any activity where food was set out on the table, be it a meal, a coffee morning or cake baking, Ronald was in there like a vulture, demolishing everything in sight. Sometimes he would collect and hide other items as well. It made him a difficult and unpopular member of the group. I suggested to staff that for the next couple of activities involving both Ronald and objects, they should try setting a precise place for him; they should draw out a square on the table, write Ronald in it, and put in the square only the objects that he needed for his part in the activity. It worked. Ronald was no longer all round the table and into everybody else's work. He confined all his activity to those objects that had been placed in his square, and became a tolerated and cooperative group member in the process.

have been called lateral thinkers, with a brain that works creatively to find quirky and unusual solutions to problems, are often the best people to pull in to this task.

A linear approach to the management of the situation described in Box 7.15 might be to decide that Ronald and objects don't mix, so they should be kept separate; Ronald should only be included in those activities where objects and food are not involved. The lateral approach went further, asking the question, 'What would Ronald be saying if he could?'. Ronald's dementia was fairly advanced; he was becoming very egocentric – in other words, turned in on himself and unable to appreciate 'otherness'. So surely he would be saying, 'Here is a plate of cakes. I like cakes, I shall eat them. Here is another plate of cakes. I like cakes, I shall eat them'. Or perhaps, 'Here are some lovely colours. I love reds and yellows and oranges. I shall have them'. Ronald has tunnel vision; he knows only his world, what he sees now, and what he wants now. Drawing the square on the table for Ronald met him where he is. He still has no appreciation of others, but he sees the square on the table with his name in it. He still knows his name. It says Ronald so it must be his; and some objects are arranged around the word Ronald, so they must be his too.

Metaphor – expressing one thing, and meaning another. Most of us have for so long been so locked into words as our foremost means of communication that we find it hard to enter this world of figure and shadow and type. But enter it we must, if ever we are to be effective in our therapeutic interventions with people who have dementia.

To date, non-verbal communication has never been perceived as a training matter for dementia care. Many dementia care trainers touch on non-verbal issues as they assist people around the intricacies of disordered behaviours, but consult any dementia care training programme, and that is all you will see – a session on 'challenging behaviours'. This is putting the cart before the horse. Challenging behaviours are but the product of non-verbal communications gone awry. If carers understood the power and the mechanics of non-verbal communications, we would be having far fewer challenging behaviours to deal with. This is far too important an issue to continue with such scant attention. Non-verbal communication needs to go on the curriculum of dementia care programmes now. Those of us who train others have a responsibility to address this issue as a matter of priority.

Key Points

- Make eye contact every time you come into contact with the person who has dementia.
- Try and ensure that you have a relaxed, friendly expression as you meet with a person with dementia.
- When you are talking or assisting with care, adopt a calm, unhurried approach. Outpacing a person can cause ill-being.
- Approach from the front and at eye level; don't invade a person's personal space without warning.
- Hand objects to a person at eye level and within six inches. Name the object, and place the person's hand on the object to help him or her start off an action if necessary (e.g. drinking tea, brushing hair).
- Adopt a running commentary to whatever you do, indicating what has just happened and what is about to happen.
- Don't talk to a colleague about a person with dementia in the presence of that person. Always include the person in your conversation.
- Validate a person's feelings/experience whenever you can; try not to get into a disagreement about facts (e.g. if a person says he or she is hungry and hasn't had breakfast, don't dispute this; offer a biscuit or banana to tide him or her over to the next meal).
- We need to be aware of the quieter, less demanding person, who often is starved of human contact. Frequent brief contacts can make an enormous difference to wellbeing.

References

Ekman P, Friesen W 1969 Non-verbal leakage and clues to deception. Psychiatry 32:85–106

Ekman P, Levenson R, Friesen W 1983 Autonomic nervous system distinguishes between emotions. Science 221:1208–1210

Goffman E 1961 Encounters: two studies in the sociology of interaction. Bobs Merrill, Indianapolis

Hall E 1966 The hidden dimension. Doubleday, New York

Hoffman S, Platt C, Barry K, Hamill L 1985 When language fails: non-verbal communication abilities of the demented. In: Hutton J, Kenny A (eds) Senile dementia of the Alzheimer type. Alan R Liss, New York

Hubbard G, Cook C, Tester S, Downs M 2002 Older people with dementia using and interpreting non-verbal behaviour. Journal of Aging Studies 16:155–167

Laing R 1967 The politics of experience. Penguin, Harmondsworth

Chapter 8

A model for dementia care

INTRODUCTION

So far in this book we have been examining the theory of occupation in dementia care, and in particular the nature of the therapeutic relationship with the dementing person. It is the purpose of this chapter now to give some structure to our thoughts on occupational practice in dementia care: the way we use and manipulate occupations in the care of the person with dementia. We make no attempt to be prescriptive – this activity for that set of circumstances. Nor are we suggesting that there is anything special about the occupations that we use in dementia care. As always we use the ordinary, the everyday, the commonplace. What we are offering is along the lines of a practice model. We are not sure whether we should call it a model, for there remains some controversy, in occupational therapy circles at least, as to what is and isn't a model. It is probably more strictly a frame of reference, expressed in the context of a schematic representation. However, it is really not terribly important how we view this schema: as a model, a frame of reference, or as something else entirely. What is important is that it should be helpful in a practical way, and serve the purpose of guiding the practitioner in the structuring of therapeutic programmes with individuals and groups. We feel that this is a beginning, a starting point, and it is our hope that over the course of time others will build upon it, amend and reshape it perhaps, as together we work towards a greater sophistication and utility.

This model (we will continue to use this term simply because it is the easiest and most descriptive) is based upon the Piagetian theory of cognitive development first discussed in Chapter 3. We have also been influenced by the developmental models of occupational therapists Ann Cronin Mosey (1981, 1986) and Claudia Kay Allen (the 'doing' section of Fig. 8.1 is adapted from Allen, Earhart & Blue's six cognitive levels, 1992). However, it would be true to say that both Mosey and Allen were also influenced by Piaget, amongst others. We have, in addition, drawn from the ideas of Donald Winnicott, whose seminal work on human development and the development of 'self' cannot be ignored.

We have attempted to put together a model which illustrates the cognitive changes that take place across the course of a dementia, and thereby the changes to an individual's ability to 'do'. Perhaps a word needs to be said, before proceeding further, about the use of stages and categories, columns and boxes. There are those who are uncomfortable about applying stages to dementia, believing this to be somehow a denial of individuality and personhood, and counterproductive to the therapeutic task. There is little logic in such a notion, though there may for some be a temptation to put people into boxes alongside the information, understanding their experience as having clearly defined parameters. We hope that our model will not be used in such a way. We use boxes for the purpose of ordering and structuring concepts, not people. The model should bend to the person, not the other way round, and we believe that this schema is sufficiently flexible to accommodate the diversity of individual experience over the course of dementia.

We like to understand the model in terms of the four developmental stages broadly described by Piaget as the reflective, the representational (we prefer the term symbolic, but the meaning is the same), the sensorimotor and the reflex. We shall address this discussion to those four headings, although it goes without saying that there are no definitive dividing lines between stages, and a considerable blurring of edges.

THE REFLECTIVE PHASE

In the young person whose cognitive development is progressing normally, this is the period of mid to late teens, characterised by a move towards mature, adult functioning. In dementia, we understand this to be that period where the first tell-tale signs of a dementing condition are starting to intrude into an otherwise healthy cognition.

Relationship to the world

Awareness of people, things and events is intact, even in the broader unseen environment represented by the individual's ability to use symbol and image. Fully developed intellectual powers and social faculties foster the capacity for self-maintenance and change, and adaptation to the vicissitudes of life in the world is a key feature. A person can bend to the influences of the environment upon him, and allow himself to change in order to accommodate them. This retention of a social awareness permits new relationships to be established, and existing relationships to continue in an equality of give and take.

Developmental stage	Reflective	Symbolic	Sensori-motor	Reflex
Stage of dementia	Early dementia	Early to middle dementia	Middle to late dementia	Late dementia
Relationship to the world	Aware of others — Alert to a broad environment — Equality in relationships — Adapts self to the world	Increasing egocentricity — Perceived environment shrinking — Increasing dependence in relationship — Assimilates world to self	→ → → →	Egocentric — Perceived environment very narrow (bubble) — Dependent upon others — World is 'me'
Thinking	Flexibility for thought — Ability to handle multiple stimuli — Deductive reasoning — Facility with language	Concrete thinking — One stimulus at a time — Lack of direction in thinking — Language impairment — Increased reliance upon symbol	↑ ↑ ↑ ↑	Little to no evidence of directed thought — Loss of language — Little or no evidence of symbol use

Doing *Key feature

	Planned actions	Exploratory actions	Goal-directed actions	Manual action	Postural actions	Automatic actions
Key feature	* Speculation and planning new courses of action	* Learning new ways of doing things	* Compliance	* Interest	Ability to move body in space (stand/walk/righting response)	Inability to stand/sit upright
				Use of hands to manipulate objects	Reflex action on objects (grasping/sucking/avoidance)	No action on objects
			Features of objects distinguished	Objects distinguished		
	Anticipation of secondary effects of actions on objects	Exploration of effects of own actions on objects	Effects of actions on objects noted	Effects of actions on objects not full perceived/understood	* Comfort	* Association between sensory cue and motor action
	Synchrony of sequencing	Ability to alter sequences according to choice	Sequencing of actions through known steps	Sequencing of actions poorly understood/carried out		
	Planning in the absence of material objects	Ability to alter actions on tools according to choice	Understanding of tool use evident	Elementary tool use evident		
	Self-directed learning	Learning by trial and error	Learning new actions by rote			

Nature of activity	Goal-directed — Rule-orientated — Competition — Co-operative group	Increasingly inappropriate — Parallel group — Increasingly related to symbol	Imitative and reflexive — Circular and repetitive — Sensori-motor — Solitary/one-to-one	↑ ↑ ↑ ↑

Activity	Games, Sports, Quizzes	Discussions, Craft, End-product tasks	Music, Dance, Art	Movement, Drama, Pottery	Spiritual, Reminiscence, Story-telling	Festive	Movement, Massage, Cooking, Rummaging	Stacking, Dolls and soft toys, Balls/bubbles/balloons, Exercise	Snoezelen, Gardening, Folding, Clowning	Singing, Rocking, Holding, Squidging	Non-verbal communication, Smiling, Stroking, Cuddling

Figure 8.1 A developmental model of practice for dementia care.

Thinking

The power of deductive reasoning is the most notable feature of a mature cognition: the flexibility to handle numbers of stimuli at once, the ability to weigh one proposition with another, to select this idea and discard that notion. Facility with language in which to convey this richness and complexity of mental processing to the world around is a complementary skill.

Doing

Doing is inextricably linked to thinking in this phase, and is characterised by planned actions, actions in which many component parts are set in sequence. Known sequences are understood and new sequences may be explored. The flexibility of thinking which characterises this stage permits changes to be made to existing relationships between actions, and between actions and objects, and facilitates the creation of new relationships. Learning is self-determined and self-directed.

Nature of activity

The type of activity predominantly engaged in by those with cognitive faculties intact is both goal-directed and rule-oriented. There is invariably a goal, an end-in-view; a person has the ability to retain that goal in his inner vision, to make plans, and to effect actions and employ objects which will enable him to move towards that goal. Rules also will often dominate activity at this stage, although they may be more commonly understood as methods or procedures or patterns. They are nevertheless rules – specified ways of doing things. Memory and comprehension are intact, and rules are therefore retained and understood, and used to structure and drive actions. Where such activity is carried out with other people, it will often be in the context of a cooperative group setting, where it is the interdependency of the parties involved which determines the achieving of the goal. Competition is often a feature of the cooperative group setting, and can contribute an additional dimension of zeal and zest in the drive towards attaining the goal.

Possible activities

Any activity which fulfills the criteria outlined above has potential for inclusion at this stage. Structured crafts which follow a pattern or a set of instructions are appropriate, such as a knitted garment, a soft toy, painting by numbers or a wooden bird table. Tasks perceived as more 'work' oriented also fit the bill: for example, typing a letter, doing the washing up, getting the shopping, building a wall. Games and sports also operate in the context of goals and rules, and have the added components of cooperative interaction and competition. There are the 'head-to-head' games of chess, draughts and snooker; small group games of Monopoly, cards and Scrabble; and games with a potential for larger group participation such as darts and bowls and party games of all sorts. The variety of course is almost endless. Quizzes also may be embraced under this heading, as may discussions. The rules governing discussions may be less evident and more informal than in a game, but they are there nevertheless: rules (usually unwritten) about leadership and turn-taking and sequencing, without an understanding of which chaos is likely to ensue. Goals too are often less clear – to convey information, to solicit opinion, to resolve argument – but still an integral feature.

It is important to note at this point that activities which we have categorised under 'earlier' developmental stages, i.e. the symbolic, the sensorimotor and the reflex, are not excluded from this reflective phase. Any of the activities listed in other phases may, of course, be welcomed by the person in early dementia. As a general rule, we might say that any activity categorised by the model at an earlier stage to the one the person is in, has a potential for therapeutic benefit. The reverse is not necessarily the case. Any activity categorised by the model at a later stage to the one the person is in has a potential to be counterproductive, perhaps even damaging. For example, a person who is in the reflective phase of a dementia may of course welcome, enjoy and derive great benefit from an activity which we have included at the sensorimotor stage, such as a massage, or a party balloon game. We all know the potential for pleasure and relaxation of activities where we don't have to think or plan. However, a person who is in the sensorimotor stage of a dementia is very unlikely to enjoy or even participate in a quiz or a game of dominoes, and attempts to encourage such a person in this direction are likely to exert pressure and induce stress; they will not be therapeutic. This is discussed in more detail below.

Examples

This section under each phase heading is designed to illustrate how a core activity may be used across all four phases of the model, with changes to accommodate it to the differing requirements of each phase. There are a number we could have chosen, but we have opted for activity related to food, activity involving music, and, perhaps because it is still a contentious issue for some people, activity using a doll.

There are a number of options related to working with food in this reflective category. One person may simply benefit from the experience of following a well-loved recipe, stage by stage, task by task; another may want to prepare a snack for a visiting relative, another to make some jam for the local fête. A cooperative element may be introduced with a group session to provide the food for a Caribbean (Thai? Scandinavian?) evening or a 'hunger lunch' for charity. A competitive dimension might be introduced in encouraging entries for the Victoria Sandwich Class at the local horticultural show.

There is a large range of possibilities for using music at this stage, from learning an instrument, to forming a small choir, to participating in a music appreciation class, to a karaoke competition.

Working with dolls in this phase could actually involve making or constructing a doll or puppet for a child or for a children's hospital or group, or possibly even putting on a puppet show; it could be in the nature of a 'dress the doll' competition for the sewing circle; or it could be the group design and building of a dolls' house to be donated to a good cause.

THE SYMBOLIC PHASE

In the child, this is a phase primarily characterised by the genesis and development of conceptual thought – in particular, of the ability to construct symbols, or mental images which relate to people or things absent from the immediate environment. The development of language is embraced in this context also. In dementia, we would understand this as a phase in which a person is becoming increasingly reliant upon symbol in mental processing, as powers of deductive reasoning diminish.

Relationship to the world

This is a phase of which a key feature is an increasing egocentricity or, as we have described it elsewhere (p. 63/64), a failure to perceive a progressively narrowing environmental field. The growing difficulty in perceiving and understanding the world of 'other' and 'out there' leads to difficulties in relationship, and to increasing dependence upon others for wellbeing and survival. The ability to adapt to external environmental influences is diminishing, and is being replaced by a delusory mechanism in which it is the world which changes. So for example, the lady whose purse is not in her handbag when she goes to look for it, is no longer able to say, 'I must have put it somewhere else; I'd better look for it' (adapting self to the world), but is quite likely to accuse the nearest other person of having stolen/removed it (assimilating world to self): 'It cannot be me, because I always keep my purse in my bag, and I have no recollection of putting it anywhere else. It must therefore be someone else'.

Piaget has suggested that in the child, this symbolic period gives way to the reflective period as the child finds more and more opportunity to satisfy needs through his inter-relationships in real life; he has less and less need of recourse to symbolic 'make-believe':

> *'In a general way it can be said that the more the child adapts himself to the natural and social world the less he indulges in symbolic distortions and transpositions, because instead of assimilating the external world to the ego he progressively subordinates the ego to reality.' (Piaget 1951)*

In our dementia care, we need to turn this statement around and recognise implicit in it the suggestion that the dementing person, unable by reason of cognitive impairment to 'subordinate the ego to reality', uses symbolic distortion and transposition to 'assimilate the external world to the ego'.

The example of Frank comes to mind. Frank, though disoriented and memory impaired, was able at one level to acknowledge his wife's death and his own admission to a residential home. However, much of the time he clearly chose to 'live' on another level, in which the residential home was The Queens (a local ballroom), where he was waiting for his wife to join him for the evening dance. He was able to acknowledge that on this level he could be in some measure content. He was, in effect, using symbol (wife alive and waiting, and The Queens ballroom) to assimilate a harsh and unacceptable external world to the ego. He appeared at this stage to be hovering on the border between the reflective and symbolic condition. As time went by, his thinking seemed to become more entrenched, settling him ever more firmly in the symbolic. We would suggest that this proposition accounts also for the innumerable episodes of 'Mother will be waiting for me' and 'I must get home to get dinner for the boys', that are so familiar to every dementia carer.

Thinking

Thinking is becoming increasingly 'concrete', inflexible and fragmented. The number of stimuli that can be accommodated in the course of mental processing is reduced, and the ability for sustained and focused thinking is declining. Language difficulties appear, and reflect disordered thought processes. There is an increased reliance upon symbol and 'fantasy' as higher critical powers diminish.

Doing

'Doing' in the symbolic phase tends to reflect the lack of flexibility evident in the cognitive realm. The ingrained actions of long-standing habits and routines and tool use are retained. Familiar objects will, by and large, be used and handled appropriately. But this is a phase which is characterised by a retreat from newness and complexity. Learning is possible (and demonstrable), but only through constant repetition, over and over again.

Nature of activity

Those principles which govern the activity of the previous, reflective phase are becoming increasingly inappropriate as a dementia progresses. The cognitive faculties required to hang on to future goals, and to make sense of sets of rules and procedures, are declining. There is therefore a need to look away from activities which are so driven. Competition also needs careful handling here. It may still, in some circumstances, provide a healthy buzz to an activity, but we need to beware of pitting somebody against his own dwindling abilities, and setting him up for failure. The quiz is a good example of an activity which can be (and often has been) misused in such a way – we need to be absolutely sure that we are not reinforcing a person's self-awareness of cognitive losses. It is only too easy to do.

As the social world of the person in this phase begins to fracture, the group setting which relies upon cooperative interaction for its function becomes increasingly inappropriate. Socialising naturally continues to be important, but we might expect that a parallel group setting will now be more comfortable for the person whose social skills are declining. A parallel group, such as the reminiscence group or the knitting circle, provides opportunity for sociality, without the demand or expectation of interaction. People can be together, without having to work together, and the group will function with or without any given individual.

The key to understanding therapeutic activity at this stage is that it is increasingly related to symbol. If, as suggested above, a person is sufficiently cognitively impaired that they are using symbolic distortion and transposition to assimilate the external world to the ego, then maybe we need to give credence to the world of fantasy in a way that we have not done before. Traditionally pragmatic, occupational therapists may have some difficulty with such a notion, but it is nevertheless an idea which merits attention. Cox (see Chapter 5) attributes great weight to the value of fantasy in human survival, seeing it as essentially a creative mechanism which facilitates adaptation, innovation and change. It is not hard to see the delusional talk and behaviour of dementia in such a light: that it is a creative way of surviving, of accommodating the loss and damage of cognitive impairment. Such in fact is the basic theory underpinning Naomi Feil's validation therapy; indeed her alternative title was 'fantasy therapy', though this is not commonly used (Feil 1982). The essential principle of such an approach then, is that practitioners should actively address and explore the 'fantasy' statement or action, acknowledging its survival function and understanding its creative drive. This may be a new departure for many practitioners, but it must be addressed if we are serious about the wellbeing of our clients with dementia.

Possible activities

Activities which we might describe as symbolic are those which have the power both to evoke inner pictures or images, and to permit a freedom of creative expression. If Frank (above) had clearly chosen to live in a world of image and fantasy, maybe our therapeutic responsibility should have been to enable him to extend that world as far as possible, in his inner life, and in the way he expressed himself outwardly. Maybe we should have made the dining room into the Queens ballroom from time to time; maybe we should have held him close and danced the last waltz; maybe we should have played 'their' tune. I don't recall that anyone ever did. I for one was too concerned about reality-orientating him at the time. But I suspect that had we done so, we would have brought some pockets of sunlight into a grey and sombre experience.

A word here about reality orientation, or, as it has recently been re-packaged, cognitive stimulation therapy (Spector et al 2003). Don't dismiss it. Learning and relearning is still possible at this stage of dementia. Sensitive, carefully individualised reality orientation techniques can improve function and wellbeing, and may be appropriate. Mrs Andrews was a lady with significant memory and language impairments (Perrin 1996). She was well into a symbolic phase, yet retained a remarkable insight into her condition, and managed to communicate this. Together, we used a reality orientation technique to 'work on' her memory. There was a small though significant improvement to her memory function, and an immense leap in her self-esteem and wellbeing – a very worthwhile intervention. However, the symbolic phase is the latest point at which reality orientation will be effective. Once a person is moving in the direction of the sensorimotor phase, it is redundant.

Any activity which centres on music, dance and movement might be considered symbolic. We have only to think of those pieces of music past and present which we make uniquely 'ours', to understand. Even a few notes, a movement, a dance step, a gesture, have the power to release images of people and places, times and occasions, and to put us in touch with our emotions in a way that no other type of activity can. Drama and story-telling have a similar potential, as has direct reminiscence work, of course. Many of these activities can and do take place in dementia care settings on a fairly unskilled, ad hoc basis. However, the development of the complementary therapy field over the last decade has offered a welcome new initiative in this area, and the potential for a major contribution of specialist expertise. We have in the past tended to look upon such therapies as luxuries: nice to have if you can afford it, but not essential to the stuff of everyday living. It is possible that we are soon going to have to revise our opinion. With their roots in the spiritual, the emotional and the elemental, and their expression in the creative, they appear ideally framed for the exploration and validation of that which we all too often dismiss as confused behaviour. These therapies need further research in dementia care.

The plastic arts – painting, pottery and sculpture in all their shapes and forms – also have a symbolic root. Here we are not talking about how to paint a still life, or how to make an ash-tray, but about that type of artistic activity which expresses itself in unstructured, free-form ways. The material is used according to the individual's own unique skills, in expressing this image or idea, that emotion or message.

Festive occasions and seasonal events also have a very special contribution to make to the symbolic phase, anchoring us in the present by their affirmation of the past. We have already noted in Chapter 5 the importance of festivity to health and wellbeing.

Lastly, we should not forget spiritual/religious activity, which is of course symbolic activity par excellence. There is today in care settings for older people, a much greater awareness of, and attention to, spiritual need, than there has been in the recent past. This is to be welcomed, for we should not think that spiritual experience dies along with the higher powers of reasoning; perhaps we could argue that it might even be richer without their intrusion. With its root in the symbolic, it is eminently possible for an act of worship to take place even quite late in the course of a dementia.

Examples

Food can be and is, of course, commonly used to great symbolic effect in many care settings, and we should make much of such opportunities. Eating is, for most people, a pleasure which abides, and will attract where other activities will not. The Halloween pumpkin, the simnel cake at Easter, the Christmas pudding, the communion bread and wine, all have that anchoring power which we have referred to above, and that evocative quality to elicit image, emotion and memory.

Music in this phase would not be used with the cerebral overtones of the reflective phase. There are two ways we might want to consider using it in this symbolic period. First, music and verse lie very deep within long-term memory, and are retained late into dementia. So we will want to make good use of that which is familiar: the Sunday hymn, the carol at the Christmas concert, or the war-time favourite in the reminiscence session. But we might also want to experiment a little with different kinds of music and sound. We are only too familiar with those musical experiences which affect our emotions and our fantasy life. Why should it be any different for the person with dementia? Such a person may well not be able to tell us what they like, or how they are affected by a particular sound or tune, but if we are sensitive and observant, we can discover much. Music and sound is such a rich resource; let us experiment with whale song, birdsong, pan pipes, the sound of a children's playground, African drumbeat, etc., etc., and discover that which makes a person smile and weep and move and dance.

In this symbolic phase we might want to make use of a doll, or a range of dolls and/or teddy bears, in the context of a reminiscence session. I still have my teddy bear. It sits on a shelf, grubby and balding, and I never look at it from one year to the next. But if someone were to ask me about it, I could enjoy recounting its history in great detail, from the extremely bad haircut I gave it at the age of about six, of which evidence still remains, to the tragic loss of growl subsequent to its first and only bath in nineteen-fifty-something. Such things are powerfully evocative. Alternatively, we might want to use a doll in the context of story-telling or drama, as an object to gather attention, as a visual aid to move the narrative along. There are many possibilities. A little creativity will broaden our perspective.

THE SENSORIMOTOR PHASE

Piaget has suggested that the practice play (the repetitive 'doing') of the sensorimotor period gives way to symbol as thought is gradually established and becomes more fluid. In dementia, we have a circumstance in which thought is becoming progressively more concrete and impoverished, and we might therefore suggest that as a dementia advances, even symbolic activity is gradually lost, and a person is left with only a most primal level of function – the sensorimotor condition.

Relationship to the world

A person in this phase of a dementia is moving (or has moved) to a position where they are experiencing the world (as far as we can tell) only in terms of their physical capacities, that which can be assimilated via the six sensory mechanisms. Awareness of people and things and events in the environment around is now very limited, and it is very much as though the person is living in a small glass bubble. There is little active contribution to relationship, and an increasingly helpless dependence upon others for the meeting of survival needs.

Thinking

There is now little evidence of directed thought. There may be some evidence of symbol use apparent in emotional or actional responses to stimuli, but little language of any real utility with which to convey either thought or image. There may be remnants of speech, and there will probably be noises of some kind.

Doing   A person in this phase is still able to 'do' – that is, to instigate actions, and to handle and use objects and tools – but is moving towards a 'doing without understanding'. So there may remain an ingrained ability to feed oneself with a spoon or to catch a ball (almost a cerebellar skill), but no comprehension that a spoon might also be used for stirring tea or taking medicine or digging up weeds, or that someone who throws you a ball invariably wants you to throw it back again. The ability to sequence complex, multi-component actions has gone, and there appears to be comfort and pleasure in limited, one-step actions which can be repeated over and over.

Piaget has described the simple, one-step, repetitive exercise of the child, performed out of its usual context for pleasure, and has suggested that this arises whenever a new skill is required, the pleasure deriving from 'being the cause'. He gives the example of the three-month-old who derives huge enjoyment from throwing his head backwards from an upright position. The behaviour started via exploration (interest in the external result) but became play (done for its own sake, for sheer pleasure). He describes also the child who discovers the possibility of making toys attached to the top of her cot swing. At just over three months this was carried out with studied interest. From four to eight months, it was never indulged in 'without a show of great joy and power'. Behaviours common to this class are throwing, pushing, pulling, filling, emptying, shaking, rubbing. Piaget notes that each new specific behaviour will eventually flag as saturation point is reached, but that, as this type of activity can reappear with each new acquisition, it can last far beyond childhood.

It is interesting to speculate on how far this might be understood as a picture of advanced dementia, for we are only too aware of how people in late dementia often engage in highly repetitive behaviours such as rubbing, picking, rocking, stroking. It may be that this is a return to a primordial form of exploration or stimulus-seeking. It is possible that we might understand the two as one and the same thing, or at least emanating from the same need source: that is, satiation of, or boredom with the current stimulus level and type. Or it may simply be that for a person whose skills are so radically depleted, single repeated actions offer a comfortable or comforting no-demand engagement with 'other'. There seem to be two types of repetitive, rhythmical actions in late dementia: that which induces pleasure and satisfaction, and that which doesn't. Ernest (see Box 6.5) was rhythmically spooning imaginary plum crumble into his mouth with every appearance of satisfaction, whilst Elsa's (see Box 6.2) repetitive 'My daddy oooh' had a different quality about it; it almost felt like a last-ditch attempt to say, 'I am alive. I must be alive, because I can hear myself making this noise. Please notice me'. Only the direct observation of the individual can guide us here.

Before we leave this section, we need just make reference once again to the use of objects at this level, and to give some consideration to what Winnicott (1951) has called 'transitional objects'. The young child who is starting to make that move of separation from mother will invariably attach himself to an object of some kind, a toy or a piece of cloth or some such, without which, it seems, he cannot exist. The object goes everywhere with him, it must always be to hand, it must never be washed, for that would change the essential character of the object and therefore of his relationship with the object. Winnicott has suggested that this transitional object is a first indication of relationship with the world, the first 'not-me' possession, and is expressly designed to assist the child in his repudiation of mother en route towards independence. We would want to suggest that some people with dementia, in their return towards dependence, often make use of an object in such a way. We need to be alert to our client's need for a toy, or a particular cardigan, or any other object which must be constantly at his side, for it may well be that this object is also a transitional phenomenon, assisting the person in his journey across an increasing dependence towards a renewed need for 'mother'. It should perhaps be a signal to us that our client is preparing for that time when he must put himself into the hands of another for his survival and care and nurture.

Nature of activity

Bearing in mind the constraints upon actions described above, we need here to confine our activities to those having a strong sensorimotor impact: in other words those activities which encourage movement, and which impinge upon all six sensory modalities. Activities which can be broken down into one-step component parts, activities which have a rhythmic, repetitive quality, are those which are usually the most comfortably received.

Possible activities

Motor activities such as the exercise group, movement to music and dance, all have these rhythmic, repetitive qualities and are entirely appropriate here. Folding tasks (towels, paper napkins), stacking tasks (chairs, boxes), dusting, wiping, polishing and sweeping, are all one-step actions repeated over and over. The product of such activity, as we saw in Chapter 6, is likely to be of little consequence; the process, for the person in the sensorimotor period, can be very rewarding. Rummaging too, is a similar process, but has an exploratory component, and is often well-used by the person who is restless, or who has a curiosity about objects. Any good unit should have a rummage box, filled with all manner of things which have 'fiddle potential', curiosity value and sensory appeal. Not being based in any one spot, I have two rummage bags. One is a tool bag full of bits of engine, old tools, things which screw together, things which pull apart. The other contains ribbons and bows, a feather boa, a bath puff, baby bootees, a large koosh ball, a loofah and numerous other assorted items. Anything goes; they don't appeal to everybody, but for some they offer a pleasurable and absorbing half-hour.

Activities which appeal predominantly to the senses are important. Massage is much under-used, but is low-demand and has an immense potential for improving wellbeing. The Snoezelen or multisensory environment offers a range of interesting sensory experiences, and has been shown to have some beneficial effects. Gardening of course has considerable sensory (as well as motor) potential, as does cooking (see below); both have tasks which can be broken down into the smallest of component parts, and fitted to individual need. Games which use balls, balloons and bubbles can have enormous appeal for many people at this stage of dementia, as indeed can dolls and soft toys. We need to think again of those things which engage and give pleasure to the child at this developmental stage, for all the reasons given in the preceding chapters; playing and playfulness comes into its own at this stage more than at any other. Children need boldness, colour, vibrancy and spontaneity; they laugh at the physically incongruous, are delighted by visual stimulus, are intrigued by tactile stimulus. There is considerable empirical evidence for the benefits of dolls and toy animals; we need to consider how we might work more creatively in this direction. The possibilities are immense – another area ripe for research.

Examples   Food needs to be used rather differently in this phase to how it is used in others, and can be exploited for its sensory properties. A colleague once shared an idea she had for a 'fruit salad group'. She gathered a number of people around a large range of different fruits on the kitchen table, and together they prepared a fresh fruit salad. The potential for sensory impact in terms of colour, shape, texture, scent and taste, is considerable. The batch of scones or marzipan fruits can offer similar opportunities.

Music and singing in this phase may make rather more of a demand upon us than in other phases, for it is likely that we will have to bury any self-consciousness and get in there and sing with the client. Our aim is for the client to obtain pleasure from the sensory impact of singing, and we may well need to encourage singing along to the music, or humming to a rhythmical movement. Crimmens (1997) has had considerable success using a microphone, enabling people to hear themselves, probably for the first time, in an unusual and dramatic way. There is also available on the market a sound and light board, a piece of apparatus with coloured lights which flash in response to voice stimulus through a microphone. We have not observed these in use in dementia settings, but they might be worth some exploration.

Many people in this phase of a dementia find great pleasure in attachment to a doll or a soft toy: holding it, cuddling it, talking to it, sleeping with it. It is our belief that we need to encourage attachments which give such comfort and warmth. But we can probably make much more of these things. Bernard Heywood, in 'Caring for Maria' (1994), found that playing the clown had a considerable impact upon his friend in the latter stages of her dementia:

> 'I've also devised a new aid to good relations and her wellbeing by making her laugh. This is achieved by indulging in antics – acting, gesticulating and walking in odd ways as one would with a child, or indeed like a real comic doing a routine. So far it's been very helpful. These antics remained helpful on and off for a considerable time, and my repertoire increased. It included wearing one or two comic, or comically arranged hats, and odd ways of dressing. Just as she could cry excessively, Maria could also laugh excessively.'

Perhaps we can draw on this, and suggest that we need to be a little bolder about losing inhibitions in this area. We are all familiar with the delight of young children at the clown and the puppet, at dressing up, at make-believe. If our return to childhood analogy holds, why should it be any different for the older person with dementia? This is uncharted territory in dementia care; maybe we need to take some risks and do some exploration.

THE REFLEX PHASE

This is the condition of late dementia, that stage which has sometimes been called vegetative, and is analogous in our model to the condition of early childhood.

Relationship to the world

We perhaps cannot strictly speak of a relationship to or with the world in this phase, because the person with dementia is now moving towards a point in which there is little or no separation between person and world. Each is an integral part of the other. We might say that 'the world is me' – in Piaget's terms he has become egocentric. In Winnicott's terms he does not know where he ends and the world begins, and vice versa.

> 'To begin with the baby does not feel himself to be separate from the environment: insofar as it is possible to talk about a self at all there is no difference between what is "me" and what is "not-me". No object external to the self is known.' (Davis & Wallbridge 1987)

We would suggest that the person with dementia is moving the same way: that he is now largely experiencing the world in the context of his reflexes to stimuli.

Piaget (1953) proposed that the consistent use of the reflex action in the child is the genesis of all future development:

> 'Almost since birth, therefore, there is "behaviour" in the sense of the individual's total reactions and not only a setting in motion of particular or local automatizations only interrelated from within. In other words, the sequential manifestations of a reflex such as sucking are not comparable to the starting up of a motor used intermittently, but constitute an historical development so that each episode depends on preceding episodes and conditions those that follow in a truly organic evolution.'

Piaget (1951) observed that the reflex, be it sucking, grasping, crying, vocalisation, is an immediate autogenetic precursor to imitation, a fundamental feature of the cognitive development process, the attempt of the child at accommodation to the external world. He believes that this is where psychology begins. We believe that in dementia care, it is also where it ends, and we should not dismiss such primitive manifestations of relations with the world from our appreciation of the experience of the person with dementia.

Thinking

This is a world pretty well closed to us at this stage of dementia. It is likely that even speech and noises have now disappeared, and there is little outward evidence of thought or intentionality. And yet how many of us have on occasion turned to that speechless person in the recliner chair, and been held by an intense unflinching gaze of the deepest communion. One can only feel at such a time that there remains until the last an unfathomable 'knowingness'. All other forms of making contact might have gone, but, as Ignatieff (see p. 52) has suggested, 'being' still remains.

Doing

As we must adjust our ideas of 'relationship' with the world in this phase of dementia, so too we need to reconsider our notions of 'doing'. 'Doing' in all other contexts so far discussed has been related to purpose and intentionality. It is not so related here. There remains the ability to move the body in space, and to interact with objects, but such interaction is now in a reflex manner only. Lastly even these reflex movements will disappear, and all that is left are random neurological signs.

Nature of activity

All is not lost, however, while reflex responses are still evident. When other forms of approach to a person are denied us because of their severe impairment, we need to consider the eliciting of reflex and imitation. For example, most carers, when wanting to encourage their client or relative to evacuate the bladder in an appropriate place at an appropriate time, are very familiar with the ploy of turning the wash-basin tap on. For whatever reason, the sound of running water can very often influence the bladder reflex, and elimination occurs. Whether this is strictly imitation, or what Piaget would call merely contagion, is for us probably neither here nor there. What is important is that it usually works. We need to consider very seriously what we bring to our interactions here, for we are wanting to encourage imitative and reflexive action, and there is every reason to expect that we will get back what we give. Are we smiling as we come to engage with the person in this latter phase? This is important to consider, for there is good evidence to suggest that changes in facial expression elicit emotion-specific activity in the autonomic nervous system (Ekman et al 1983). Zajonc et al (1989) have conducted a fascinating series of experiments which demonstrate that even the mere arranging of one's facial features into the form of a smile (without any underpinning emotion) is sufficient to improve wellbeing in a small measure. This is important information. A person with dementia may not know why he is smiling, but until we know otherwise, maybe the mere fact that he *is* smiling, albeit in imitation, is reason to believe that his wellbeing is in some measure increased.

When doing has ceased, all we are left with is the possibility of our own 'doing to' our client, and this is where we need to give serious consideration to the notion of mothering as an important concept for final stage dementia care (see Chapter 10).

Possible activities

It is perhaps more appropriate in this phase to speak of actions rather than of activities. For in a sense a person is now only able to engage in the component parts of activities.

Ida was a lady in the earlier part of this final phase of dementia. She could sit upright, and make noises, and just about hold a cup, and that was about the extent of her 'doing'. Nobody knew how much she could see or how much she could hear. I sat with her one afternoon, put my hand on hers in case she should wish to take it, and attempted to respond to some of her noises, reflecting what I felt were the tones that she was using. At one point I said to her, 'Tell me about it, Ida'. She did. Coincidence or whatever, she leant forward and out poured a stream of excited vowel sounds which went up and down and on and on. She had my hand in a vice-like grip, though this did not feel like affection – more like a random clasping of emotional intensity; it could have been the arm of the chair. When she had finished speaking, for that is undoubtedly what it was for her, she took my hand to her mouth and started to gnaw my knuckles enthusiastically. She gnawed for a long time. It is perhaps fortunate that she had no teeth.

I have no idea what this interlude meant for Ida, but it felt very positive. She clearly had no real concept of me as a person; I was a sound to respond to, an object to clutch, a bone to gnaw upon. But it was nevertheless an engagement with the world, and insofar as any outsider could judge, it felt as though it had to be a lot more satisfying than her usual hours spent staring vacantly into space.

It is possible to sustain communication at some level quite late into most dementias, and we need to make good use of those non-verbal mechanisms which are open to us. Where there is still some 'doing' left we need to encourage imitation and reflection of our own. We need to smile, to sing, to respond to noises, to stretch and encourage people's own movements. If they are still able to feed themselves in any way, shape or form, we need to make every effort to facilitate that; and if that means squidgy food and spilt tea, it doesn't matter. It is initiative; it is engagement with the world, and should be fostered.

Where 'doing' has all but ceased, we can only 'do to'; we need to take our model from the mothering of early childhood, and become comfortable with rocking and stroking, holding and cuddling. These are the needs of the newborn. We believe they are also the needs of the person in the final stages of dementia.

Examples

Some people at this stage will still be able to feed themselves, and we would hope that practitioners will still be able to appreciate the tactile value of food in this phase, messy though it may be. If it is important for the child at this developmental stage to feed himself and get covered with egg and soggy toast at the same time, then it is important for the person with dementia, and we need to resist the temptation to have a quick chin-wipe every five minutes. Of course we need to clean up at the end; we do not leave our toddler with congealed food all over his clothes. But for the duration of the meal, our client needs to be as self-determining as possible. A colleague with whom I once carried out a dementia care-mapping exercise, observed a lady at the breakfast table. Breakfast was long finished, but the table had not been cleared, and the lady either couldn't or didn't wish to leave. She spent the better part of an hour 'walking' her toast crusts up and down the table, with every appearance of absorption and satisfaction.

Can we engage people in this stage of dementia in song? Probably not; but we can engage them in noises, and we can – if we can dispense with our inhibitions – sing *to* them. We do not know what remains, and what we sing may well not be recognised, but there is something elemental in the rhythm of song, and we have every reason to believe that this might be comforting and pleasurable.

We have already spoken of the transitional object above. If there is no evidence of a doll or a toy or any other significant object, we believe that it is a good practice for something to be offered. It might be rejected or ignored; that is not important – what is important is that we provide an opportunity for attaching to something that will assist, comfort and ease the journey towards absolute dependence.

The key to using this model, of course, is an understanding of where the person with dementia might be placed within the schema. This is a matter which will be decided in part on the basis of clinical experience, and in part on an accurate assessment of a client's ability to think and to do. This is addressed in the next chapter.

Key Points

- It is helpful to perceive dementia, and therapeutic intervention in dementia, under four headings, each of which reflects a level of cognitive development.
- There are clear changes over the course of a dementia, in one's perception of, and relationship to the world, and in the ability to think and to do.
- Activities may be broadly divided into classes which in some measure 'match' cognitive ability.
- The notion of 'matching' activity to cognitive level is a helpful guideline, but not to be considered in any way prescriptive.
- A general rule of thumb for the selection of appropriate activity is that most people will derive benefit from an activity which matches their level of cognitive ability, or which is at an earlier developmental level. The reverse is not the case; most people who engage in an activity which matches a later developmental level than their own, will find the activity stressful and counterproductive.
- In late dementia, we need to recognise that actions rather than activities are the focus of intervention.
- It can be helpful to understand the engagement in activity over the course of a dementia, as a journey in which doing is gradually relinquished to being.

References

Allen C, Earhart C, Blue T 1992 Occupational therapy treatment goals for the physically and cognitively disabled. American Occupational Therapy Association, Rockville, MD

Crimmens P 1997 Storymaking and creative groupwork with older people. Jessica Kingsley, London

Davis M, Wallbridge D 1987 Boundary and space: an introduction to the work of D W Winnicott. H Karnac, London

Ekman P, Levenson R, Friesen W 1983 Autonomic nervous system distinguishes between emotions. Science 221:1208–1210

Feil N 1982 Validation: the Feil method. Edward Feil Productions, Cleveland, OH

Heywood B 1994 Caring for Maria. Element Books, Shaftesbury

Mosey A 1981 Occupational therapy: configuration of a profession. Raven Press, New York

Mosey A 1986 Psychosocial components of occupational therapy. Raven Press, New York

Perrin T 1996 Problem behaviour and the care of elderly people. Winslow Press, Oxon

Piaget J 1951 Play, dreams and imitation in childhood. Routledge and Kegan Paul, London

Piaget J 1953 The origin of intelligence in the child. Routledge and Kegan Paul, London

Spector A, Thorgrimsen L, Woods B 2003 Efficacy of a cognitive stimulation therapy programme for people with dementia: randomized controlled trial. British Journal of Psychiatry 183:248–254

Winnicott D 1951 Transitional objects and transitional phenomena. In: Winnicott D (1958) Collected papers: through paediatrics to psycho-analysis. Tavistock, London

Zajonc R, Murphy, Inglehart M 1989 Feeling and facial efference: implications of the vascular theory of emotion. Psychological Review 96(3):395–416

Chapter 9

Assessing capacity for doing and promoting engagement

INTRODUCTION

I remember clearly a conversation I once had with a professional colleague in a long-term care setting. We were discussing Jim, who was in the process of being assessed. Jim was a strong-willed but very polite and likeable person. He had been diagnosed with vascular dementia, in addition to arthritis which limited his mobility. I had observed him eating his lunch earlier and seen that he was struggling to use the cutlery that he had been given. I was interested to know, as part of my assessment, how he coped with self care activities on the ward. 'Well', said my colleague, 'he manages quite well but he needs a lot of help and takes forever … the problem is he's just very lazy'.

More about Jim later; the point here is that my colleague's attitude was the result of a lack of understanding about how dementia can affect a person's capacity for 'doing', and back then during the 1990s, this gap in knowledge was widespread. Our perception is that knowledge about occupation and capacity for 'doing' in the field of dementia care has improved dramatically, both within the profession of occupational therapy and throughout the care industry generally.

In this chapter we look first at an ethical rationale for ensuring good occupational practice in dementia care and at how a broader understanding about occupation and different kinds of 'doing' is important for this. In the second part of the chapter we focus in detail on Allen's cognitive disabilities model (1985) which provides a framework for understanding *capacity for doing* and how this changes during the course of dementia. Finally we discuss the tools we have used to profile wellbeing as an outcome measure of a good occupational approach.

AN ETHICAL BASIS

Before moving on to define and discuss capacity for doing, we propose an ethical framework within which occupational interventions can be justified. This is especially important for people who have dementia, who may struggle to communicate easily their consent to or opinion about the actions of others or the activities that they may find themselves being asked to take part in.

It goes without saying that society trusts care providers to act in the best interests of the people they care for. They are trusted to be responsible holders of the caring *role*. This is an important distinction from that of being trusted to perform particular *tasks*. For example, it is not simply the giving of injections (a medical task) that society trusts doctors to do. Society trusts the doctor to act professionally in the doctor role. Giving an injection is not always beneficial for the patient, and society trusts the doctor, as part of the doctor role, to know who should be given and who should not be given an injection.

In the same way, it is not simply the task of running 'activities' that society trusts care providers to do. Rather, it is the provision of a day to day living experience (and joining in with activities may be part of that) which promotes or maintains physical and/or mental wellbeing. This is why the performance of 'tasks' in isolation, for example running an exercise group, can be potentially irresponsible. Part of the care provider's role is to understand and justify whether the tasks performed serve the overall purpose or aim, and this requires a certain knowledge base. Just as the task of giving an injection is sometimes not in the interests of the patient, the task of providing an activity, such as an exercise group, does not necessarily serve the purpose of promoting wellbeing.

We suggest the rationale in Figure 9.1, derived from the work of the philosopher Twiss (1977), which we offer to dementia care providers as a foundation for constructing a responsible occupational approach in dementia care.

Therapeutic interventions refer to specific tasks undertaken by the care provider. In dementia care, these might include tasks such as giving help with personal care, playing a game or reminiscing or assisting a person during a meal time.

Therapeutic aims are connected with the care provider's function within the larger social and institutional fabric of life. In modern day dementia care, the aims of care provision are less custodial and medical in style, giving equal weight to human social and psychological needs. The Commission for Social Care Inspection in the UK (CSCI 2007) has recently published a new outcomes framework for adult social care. The seven outcomes are: improved health and wellbeing; improved quality of life; making a positive contribution; exercise of choice and control; freedom from discrimination or harassment; economic wellbeing; and personal dignity and respect.

Figure 9.1 A therapeutic rationale.

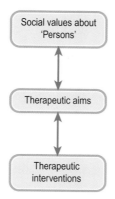

Today's care providers then, have a much broader remit and as in the example of the doctor's injection, the provision of care tasks such as feeding people, cleaning people or providing activities do not in themselves necessarily meet any therapeutic aim (or CSCI outcome). So for example, in helping a person with eating, the care provider should be looking for adaptations to the eating process or the environment that will make the most of the person's capacity and potential for eating and enjoying food, rather than simply finding ways to get food into the person.

Fortunately, the staff in the home where Helen was cared for (Box 9.1) were keen to learn new approaches and happily agreed to alter their responses at meal times. Now Helen uses only her fork, her food is presented in bite size pieces in a lipped plate, and she is able to enjoy the taste, smell and the look of her food as well as living her own experience of feeding herself. Finger foods are also available, and staff recognise that eating with fingers is a far more enriching experience than the one observed during the evaluation described in the above example.

Box 9.1

During a recent evaluation in a residential home, I observed a careworker trying to help Helen with her lunch. Helen was struggling to use the knife and fork that had been placed in her hands. The careworker started Helen off with the knife and fork but Helen could only manage her fork. The careworker insisted that she use the knife as well and repeatedly placed the knife back in her hand. Although Helen made a few attempts and went through the motions of pushing food with her knife once or twice, she was unable to engage in a free flowing manner with her food. Before long, Helen just 'switched off' and stared blankly into space before finally dropping off to sleep at the table. A few moments later, the careworker returned and woke Helen abruptly out of her sleep, placing the knife and fork once more into Helen's hands. Helen still couldn't manage and so the careworker took over and hurriedly spoon fed Helen herself.

We feel that it is good practice for care providers to be able, at any point in their day to day work, to be able to make the link between what they are doing (therapeutic interventions) with why they are doing it (therapeutic aims) – to be able to explain why, for example, it is a good idea for a grown adult to eat with her fingers.

Thirdly, there are *values about persons*. Modern day dementia care aims to be 'person-centred'; it requires care providers to work from a value base of equal rights and citizenship for people who have dementia; to provide individualised care based on an understanding of the perspective of the person who has dementia; and to provide care within a positive and supportive social psychology (CSCI 2007). For the future, we would like dementia care providers to be confident and comfortable in explaining what they are doing and why in relation to these values. In the example of Helen, it could be argued that her freedom of choice and the opportunity to use her own potential was being undermined by the actions of the care provider. From her perspective and in keeping with her own individual abilities, she would have engaged freely with her food in a way that her mind and body allowed her, i.e. with a fork and her fingers. Presenting her with finger foods and bite-sized food items (the therapeutic intervention) allowed her to engage in a way that utilised her capacity and potential (the therapeutic aim), and which upheld her right to have care provided in an individualised way and from her own perspective (the social or person-centred value).

This describes an ethically responsible occupational approach for dementia care providers, and knowledge about how dementia impacts on 'capacity for doing' is crucially important to identify an individualised approach that will achieve the aim of positive engagement and wellbeing.

CAPACITY FOR DOING

Generally speaking, people who do not have dementia have the capacity to do many things in different ways; to engage with people, tasks and objects without difficulty. They are in full control of their thinking and their physical abilities and can use both, in harmony, to achieve what they set out to do. Each person has a unique way of engaging with her world, and this does not change with the onset of dementia. Dementia simply complicates matters. Based on what we know of the functions of different parts of the brain, the developmental acquisition of certain abilities and the effect of environment on wellbeing (and logically then on performance), it is not surprising that people who have dementia each have their own unique way of doing.

What we offer here is drawn from a number of ideas, theories and approaches and we encourage others to participate in the ongoing work to shift thinking away from the widespread notion that having dementia equals being unable to 'do'.

When it comes to engaging with objects, and from there with activity in its broader sense, the skills of grasping objects, differentiating between different objects, sustaining action on objects and working with a goal in mind are the 'doing' skills that we acquire after birth. These skills build on to each other (see Chapter 8) making it possible for us to develop from being able just to grasp an object, such as a rattle or a spoon when we are very young, to being able to engage successfully with very complex tasks at maturity such as driving a car.

Having dementia can cause a person to lose one or more of these skills; this then renders them unable to engage with people, tasks or objects in the same way as an unimpaired person. Typically though, the person is judged 'unable' which leads to a style of care that takes over for the person or denies them manageable opportunities for engaging with the world, and which results in a negative mood state and ill-being. And so the spiral goes as negative mood state and ill-being are then understood to be part of the dementing process.

The spiral is avoidable however, if the care provider has an understanding of the many different ways of doing and can encourage and support accordingly. For example, a person who cannot differentiate objects will not be able to eat a meal using a knife and a fork, but they may be able to hold onto a spoon whilst being fed or even to manage a single eating implement or eat with fingers. To take over feeding completely greatly reduces that person's opportunities for being in their world and having some control over it. This is a good example of an intervention that does not serve a person-centred therapeutic aim.

An overview of some the different ways of engaging with what is outside of us is shown in Table 9.1. They are listed in the same order as the

Table 9.1   Different ways of engaging

Engaging with:	Engaging by:	Example
An object	Gazing	The person is looking at her bag
	Grasping	She grips the bag with her fingers
	Holding	She is keeping hold of her bag clutching it to her chest
An action or task	Manipulating	She changes the position of her bag
	Acting on	She puts it on her lap and explores the clasp
	Keeping going	She continues to explore the clasp
	Noting effects	She sees that the top of the bag opens when she moves the clasp
	Goal directed action	She opens her bag to look inside
A person	Eye contact	The person looks into the eyes of his carer
	Physical contact	He leans against his wife during her visit
	Single sound or word directed at or in response to another	He replies hello to another resident
	Verbal exchange	He has a brief conversation about his meal
	Group participation	He joins in a group quiz activity

Key:								
Low challenge engagement		++	+++	++++	+++++	++++++	+++++++	High challenge engagement

order in which they develop from babyhood, starting with ways that are less cognitively difficult or challenging and moving through ways that are progressively more challenging. The more challenging ways of engaging are much more likely to be out of range for some people who have dementia but here lies the key to our model for an occupational approach. Occupation is not something that becomes out of reach for a person who has dementia; it is rather the case that the type of occupation that the person has capacity for and therefore a drive for, changes over time from high demand to low demand. A most important principle here is that there is no such thing as being unable to 'do', and that gazing at a face or a passing shape is just as valid and potentially rewarding form of occupation as looking in a handbag or driving a car if the challenge matches the person's capacity for doing.

ENGAGING WITH OBJECTS AND TASKS

The work of Claudia Kay Allen (Allen 1985, Allen et al 1992) and later, Conroy (1996), Perrin (1997a,b), Pool (2007) and May (2008) has made an important contribution in broadening care providers' understanding about the different ways in which a person with dementia engages with objects and tasks.

Allen's Leather Lacing Assessment

Allen's Leather Lacing Assessment (Allen 1990) has provided an invaluable tool, in our experience, for gaining insight into how the person with dementia engages with objects and tasks. This test uses a simple functional task, a leather lacing task, as a screening assessment to ascertain the person's capacity for doing. Allen has proposed six levels of capacity to engage with objects and tasks (see Chapter 8 and Fig 8.1 for a schematic representation of these levels):

- Level 1 – automatic actions
- Level 2 – postural actions
- Level 3 – manual actions
- Level 4 – goal-directed activity
- Level 5 – exploratory actions
- Level 6 – planned actions.

This assessment is used by occupational therapists to assess, for instance, whether a person can grasp objects, distinguish objects, sustain action on objects, note the effects on objects and/or use all objects. It provides the therapist with an *initial* impression of how the person engages with objects. There are detailed sub-levels within each level to make distinctions between developmental benchmarks. For example at level 3.0, a person is able to grasp objects. At level 3.2 he can grasp objects and distinguish objects, at level 3.4 he can grasp objects, distinguish objects and sustain his action on objects, and so on. The therapist, having gained this initial impression, is in a position to check out its validity as she gets to know the patient better.

Here is Jim's story (to whom we referred at the beginning of this chapter), describing how his capacity for doing changed over time as his dementia progressed.

When Jim retired, he decided to use some of his savings to make an annual visit home to Ireland to visit his nephews and nieces and their families. He always travelled in the autumn but would start his planning in the spring. This involved shopping around for good deals on air fares, making telephone calls to each individual niece and nephew to plan an itinerary that suited them and didn't interfere with their work and family commitments, and then piecing everything together. He would type out a plan for each family and send it ahead of his arrival. His family in Ireland first noticed a change when, for the first year ever, he failed to send a plan. He talked, ahead of time, in general terms to each nephew and niece about his visit and gave his arrival details before he left but that was all. Only by chance, the day before he was due to arrive, did one of his nieces realise that nobody had been asked to collect Jim from the airport. She quickly organised a lift and one of her brothers collected Jim. The visit didn't go too well this time because Jim hadn't arranged with each family member how long he would be staying. Last minute plans had to be made and this caused confusion, inconvenience and sadly, two of Jim's nieces fell out over a misunderstanding about the arrangements. Nobody realised at the time, but this visit marked the onset of Jim's dementia. He was losing his capacity for *planned action*.

Jim's hobby had always been music. He loved listening to all sorts of modern and classical music. His taste and his collection were wide ranging including all of the Beatles music and much treasured old Irish folk music. He took it upon himself after retirement to make tapes for the young children in his Irish family. He wanted them to have access to the wide range of music available to him living in England. On the tapes he made for the children, he enjoyed mixing a little bit of talking with different tracks of music from his own collection. He usually managed to send one tape off to Ireland each month. About six months after his return from his holiday in Ireland, the tapes stopped.

On his retirement from the company, he was presented with a new 'Midi System' which he had postponed using. He wasn't too sure about how to rig it up. By chance he mentioned this to a neighbour who offered the help of her son to install the new system and show Jim how to operate it. Just before Christmas, the young man finally found time to call on Jim and switch the midi system for the old one. This he did very quickly before spending half an hour or so showing Jim how to use it. Jim struggled to get the hang of the new system straight away but the neighbour's son left the instruction book out for Jim and felt sure that with a little practice he would eventually be able to use the new machine.

The old hi-fi was boxed up and stored in the attic. Unfortunately Jim wasn't able to learn how to use the new midi system despite several attempts. He kept making the same mistakes over and over again. He managed sometimes to play music but not to tape it, because when he pressed the button that the neighbour's son had shown him it flashed up 'play'. Jim couldn't solve the problem, and was unable to learn that he needed to keep his finger on the button for longer to move the mode onto 'tape'. Jim didn't worry too much; he felt he was losing interest anyway in making tapes and that the children were probably old enough now to make their own if they wanted to. Jim was losing his drive and ability for *exploratory action*. This in turn was affecting his ability to learn and to solve problems and gradually, his range of activities and outings was diminishing.

Despite his struggle with planned action and exploratory action, Jim was still living successfully at home. He was still able to do routine tasks inside and outside the home in familiar environments. However, slowly, problems emerged as he failed to keep track of less routine jobs such as having his trousers and jackets dry cleaned, paying bills, having his eyes tested, visiting the dentist and keeping up his prescription for his heart tablets. His world was becoming smaller as he began to avoid new experiences such as day trips with the church group. Gradually, Jim was relinquishing certain roles such as treasurer for the church group and chairman of the local golf club. By spring the following year, he decided not to go to Ireland for his annual trip. When one of his nieces phoned, he told her that he would maybe come next year but that he couldn't afford to visit annually anymore.

Of course, these changes in Jim were very subtle. Family and friends did not notice anything amiss but Jim at times felt deeply anxious; he felt that 'something' was wrong but he couldn't put his mind to pinpointing what it was. For Jim, many aspects of daily living remained unaffected and he was still able to do some *goal-directed* activities such as day-to-day food shopping, making tea, making his bed and keeping his small garden in order.

On a very hot day that summer, while he was gardening, Jim had a heart attack and was rushed into hospital. During his recovery on the medical ward, staff noticed that he seemed disorientated and distressed. From here he was referred to the local psychogeriatric assessment ward where he was assessed using the Allen Leather Lacing Assessment at level 4.4. This indicated that he was able to act in a goal-directed fashion for familiar routines but that he needed help to attend to detail or to cope with change.

Two fellow patients on the ward had also been assessed. Janet was assessed at level 3.3; she was able to grasp objects and distinguish objects but struggled to sustain her action on objects. Bill was assessed at level 2.4; he was unable to grasp objects purposefully. He lived his life in a 'postural' fashion wanting to walk (sometimes, it seemed to others, excessively) and to move his body and parts of his body around in space. He enjoyed being mobile and pushing furniture around the ward.

Jim, Janet and Bill each needed different approaches to enjoy an occupational life. Bill responded to a playful approach. He laughed out loud when we batted a balloon backwards and forwards, and there are a number of reasons why he engaged so successfully with this activity. Cognitively, the Allen assessment indicated that, at level 2.4, he can accomplish a number of developmental benchmarks. He could withdraw from tactile stimuli and from visual stimuli. The balloon presented visual stimulation to Bill and so he responded to it as such, rather than because he necessarily recognised it as a balloon. Bill could also locate stimuli; his impulse was to turn his head to locate the stimulus, which was, in this example, the balloon.

At level 2.4 Bill was also able to rock and move from a sitting position and to raise body parts. Again, engaging with the moving balloon allowed him to exercise these abilities, and he enjoyed doing so. In terms of general mobility, Bill had enough trunk stability to stay seated in an upright position; he was also able to use righting reactions to prevent himself from falling over, and he could walk on flat surfaces. Batting the balloon back and forth, especially as it was done from a standing position, provided the opportunity for Bill to feel alive and functional and to enjoy mastery over his own body. Bill's performance in the Allen assessment indicated potential difficulty with subsequent developmental behaviours, the most immediate of these being 'directed walking'. This requires the cognitive capacity to be able to walk with a destination in mind. To stretch him then, or to probe, in the therapeutic sense, to retain what is at risk of being lost, we wanted to bat the balloon away from Bill occasionally and encourage and help him to see the balloon and to walk towards it. In this way, we were helping him to retain the ability to walk with a destination in mind. It was possible at this level that Bill might have experienced the satisfaction of 'striving in action', a state of being that, as we have already argued in earlier chapters, is fundamental for optimum health and wellbeing.

Such an approach would not have gone down well with Jim, who preferred more structured forms of engagement such as making snacks and bed making. At level 4.4, Jim had the cognitive capacity for all that Bill could do, and more. He walked with a destination in mind automatically, without having to think consciously about it. His performance in the Allen assessment indicated that he would also be able to engage, without struggling at all, in manual actions. He could grasp objects, distinguish them, sustain his actions on them and note the effects of what he did. At this level, Jim could operate in a 'goal-directed' fashion – but only to a degree. He was able to 'sequence' – that is, to direct himself through *familiar* steps in an activity to complete what he wanted to do. Jim liked bed making and other general tidying-up tasks because he could achieve them, and he experienced satisfaction from seeing that he had achieved them. His cognitive difficulties were more subtle than Bill's. Although Jim could cope with familiar sequences, he could not memorise new sequences. To reach a 'striving in action' position with Jim, we worked with him closely to help him to complete less familiar sequences such as painting a picture or trying a new recipe. The important thing for Jim was that he did not need help to engage in familiar sequences; he needed to be in an environment that allowed him to do this, and he did need help to enjoy new or different activities.

Janet liked company while she pottered. Pressure to complete tasks undermined her wellbeing; she needed an environment full of different types of objects with which to engage. Janet's performance in the Allen assessment told us that she could not, like Jim, operate in a goal-directed fashion. She could grasp objects and distinguish objects, but found it difficult to sustain her actions on objects. This is why 'pottering' was comfortable for her. While she did this, she was able to enjoy grasping objects and enjoy the difference of them without being under pressure to stay with them or achieve anything with them. It stretched her to sustain her actions; we wanted to engage in this with her from time to time, for example, helping her to continue wiping up until the plates were done, or to continue folding the towels until the pile was finished.

The Pool Activity Level instrument for occupational profiling (PAL)

An adaptation of Allen's model, the Pool Activity Level (Pool 2007) provides a practical framework for easy use by the care sector at large for developing occupational plans for people who have dementia. The PAL comprises a life history profile; a checklist of how a person carries out everyday tasks; an activity profile which assists the translation of understanding into practice; an individual action plan for personal activities of daily living; and an outcome sheet for recording results. Care providers use the tool to identify at which activity level a person is operating. There are four activity levels which reflect those identified in the model of Chapter 8: these are *planned* – orientated to obvious goals; *exploratory* – more concerned with the process of an activity than the goal; *sensory* – concerned with the impact on own senses; and *reflex* – sub-conscious responses to direct stimulation.

Capacity for doing template

More recently, a short 'capacity for doing' template has been developed (May 2008) which provides a hierarchy of 'doing skills' that the care provider can observe while a person who has dementia is eating; this helps to provide an initial idea of the person's mode of doing (as originally defined by Allen) so that activities and interventions can be planned appropriately.

We do not advise the use of these assessments or profiling tools in isolation. Having an idea about the 'mode of doing' of the person with dementia is only part of the picture and will not be enough. An enriched profiling process is recommended which also takes into account life history, health, personality, neurological impairment (see Chapter 1) and the extent to which the person's psychological, spiritual and emotional needs are being met (May 2008).

WELLBEING AND ILL-BEING

Understanding a person's capacity for doing helps us to form a plan or an approach, but we need to be sure that what has been planned is happening and that it is resulting in the desired outcome – which is improving or maintaining wellbeing.

Within a person-centred value base, the rationale is that cognitive impairment does not cause ill-being; ill-being can be prevented and wellbeing improved or maintained if a person's needs for comfort, attachment, inclusion, identity and occupation are being met (Brooker 2007). Ill-being is an experience that results when these needs are ignored and where the person becomes disengaged from doing and from the world around them generally. Cognitive decline is a single pathway among a complex structure of other streets and roads and does not inevitably lead to being lost. In short, wellbeing is within reach for all human beings with or without dementia!

The Bradford Dementia Group (2005) Well and Ill Being Profiling Tool, Dementia Care Mapping (DCM), and The Positive Response Schedule (Perrin 1997a) are three good tools for profiling the wellbeing of people who have dementia.

The Bradford Dementia Group well and ill being profiling tool

At the time of writing, the Bradford Dementia Group is revising its well- and ill-being profiling tool – a method that does not require formal training and can be used in both communal care settings and for individuals living in the community. Box 9.2 lists the indicators of well- and ill-being that make up the profiling tool. It is an instrument that care providers can use to observe and monitor how individual people with dementia are faring and can be administered by observation and/or interview. With the observation method, the care provider makes judgments about the person based on what they have seen over a period of time while caring for that person. The interview method involves asking the person directly to report on his or her own wellbeing. Working then from a profile of emotional strengths and weaknesses, care providers can develop occupational plans that aim to build on these strengths and reduce or compensate for weaknesses.

Box 9.2

The Bradford Dementia Group's Well- and Ill–being Indicators

Wellbeing indicators

1. Can communicate wants, needs & choices
2. Makes contact with other people
3. Shows warmth or affection
4. Shows pleasure or enjoyment
5. Alertness, responsiveness
6. Uses remaining abilities
7. Expresses self creatively
8. Is cooperative or helpful
9. Responds appropriately to people/situations
10. Expresses appropriate emotions
11. Relaxed posture or body language
12. Sense of humour
13. Sense of purpose
14. Signs of self-respect

Ill–being indicators

1. Tense body
2. Appears agitated, restless
3. Expresses anxiety, fearfulness
4. Appears angry/aggressive
5. Shows frustration
6. Appears depressed, in despair
7. Expresses sadness, grief
8. Appears listlessness, withdrawn
9. Expresses boredom

Risk factors for ill-being

1. Has pain, physical discomfort
2. An outsider (feels/is different to others)
3. Is easily 'walked over' by others
4. Is disliked/feared by others

Dementia Care Mapping

Dementia Care Mapping (Bradford Dementia Group 2005) provides a framework, grounded in person-centred care, for enabling practitioners and carers in group care settings to profile mood and the nature and the quality of engagement experienced by people who have dementia. A trained mapper can 'track' up to six people at any one time, recording every five minutes the mode of engagement (i.e. what the participant is doing), along with their mood state. Levels of mood and engagement use a numerical value system which ranges from –5 (very great signs of negative mood) to +5 (very happy, absorbed, engrossed). The mapper is also in a position to note all that is happening or not happening within the participant's environment. The final 'map' provides a detailed profile of the range of behaviours engaged in and the pattern of mood and engagement for each individual and the whole group. Written notes, taken by the mappers during the evaluation, provide additional useful information that is helpful for understanding what it is within the environment that has caused or triggered positive or negative mood and engagement.

Figure 9.2 shows the results of a Dementia Care Mapping evaluation for Vanda. Immediately, it can be seen that she has spent around 14% of her time in negative mood and engagement. The care provider would be led as a result of this to consider her overall wellbeing. By looking back at the raw data sheets and analysing in more detail, it would be possible to see which particular incidents related to Vanda's negative mood and engagement during the map. Care providers may want to look more closely at Vanda's experience of care and to reflect on their potential to improve matters for her. It can also be seen that Vanda has a good capacity for experiencing positive mood and engagement. A closer look at the data would provide insights into the triggers and conditions that bring this state of being about for her, with a view to improving her overall wellbeing in the care setting.

The Activity Profile for the group shown in Figure 9.3, with the codes explained below it, highlights engagement in activities such as interacting

Figure 9.2 Wellbeing profile.

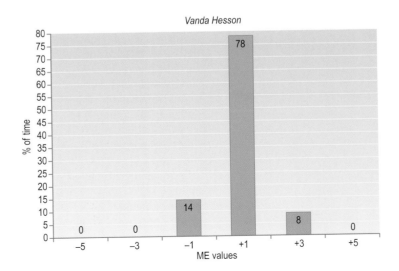

Figure 9.3 Activity profile.

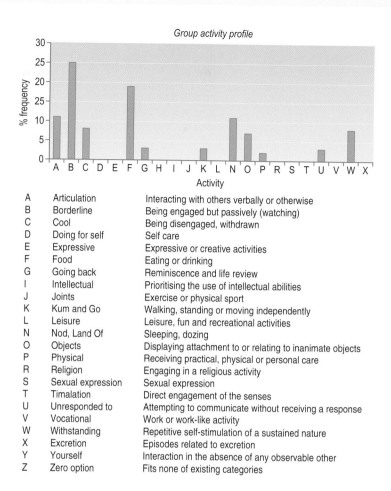

A	Articulation	Interacting with others verbally or otherwise
B	Borderline	Being engaged but passively (watching)
C	Cool	Being disengaged, withdrawn
D	Doing for self	Self care
E	Expressive	Expressive or creative activities
F	Food	Eating or drinking
G	Going back	Reminiscence and life review
I	Intellectual	Prioritising the use of intellectual abilities
J	Joints	Exercise or physical sport
K	Kum and Go	Walking, standing or moving independently
L	Leisure	Leisure, fun and recreational activities
N	Nod, Land Of	Sleeping, dozing
O	Objects	Displaying attachment to or relating to inanimate objects
P	Physical	Receiving practical, physical or personal care
R	Religion	Engaging in a religious activity
S	Sexual expression	Sexual expression
T	Timalation	Direct engagement of the senses
U	Unresponded to	Attempting to communicate without receiving a response
V	Vocational	Work or work-like activity
W	Withstanding	Repetitive self-stimulation of a sustained nature
X	Excretion	Episodes related to excretion
Y	Yourself	Interaction in the absence of any observable other
Z	Zero option	Fits none of existing categories

with others, passive social involvement and eating. The profile also clearly highlights a poverty of activity in the home evidenced by the lack of walking, games, physical exercise and such like. DCM data can be produced for both individuals and for groups and can be used to evaluate the impact of occupational or general care plans for individuals and for the group as a whole, or to inform new plans. DCM promotes a richer understanding about the necessary conditions for wellbeing and positive engagement.

Care providers involved in the provision of activities often face considerable pressure to work with groups, and there is an underlying assumption here that group activities are a good thing, that they automatically bring about wellbeing. Dementia Care Mapping has shown us that this is not always the case. Many people with dementia do not like being in groups; many people with dementia do not like organised activities; many people with dementia cannot engage in what's on offer without one-to-one help, perhaps to encourage their gaze in a helpful direction or to place an object at eye level. Boxes 9.3 to 9.6 are extracts from raw data sheets which were completed as part of an evaluation of how activities were impacting on the

Box 9.3

Notes from DCM raw data sheet: 6/5/07

11.05 Vanda is clearly not enjoying the group activity. 'Oh shut up' she mutters under her breath about the activities organiser. Three of the eight in the lounge are not engaged in the activity or with anything or anybody else at all – these people clearly need a different approach.

11.55 A marked improvement for Mrs G, who usually spends most of the day pacing up and down the corridor asking passers by if they have seen a red car. During this morning's activity session, she has remained seated and fully engaged in what has been happening.

Box 9.4

Notes from DCM raw data sheet: 21/7/07

Janet arrives in the dining room at 9.15 and her mood and engagement is good (+3). She initiates conversation with those around her and clearly enjoys her breakfast. After breakfast, she sits quietly for a while and then gets up and begins to get busy. There are no objects to touch or jobs to do in this home, and Janet is desperately looking for work to do. So, she combs her slippers, she sings beautifully with a clear rhythm and melody. This self-initiated creative expression and work-like activity maintain her wellbeing for a while, but by 11.00 she is starting to become anxious. Her sense of purposefulness is diminishing in the empty environment. Her mood and engagement degenerate to +1 and then finally to −1 by 11.30 when she is observed to be just staring into space.

Box 9.5

Notes from DCM raw data sheet: 3/3/07 a.m.

At 11.40 Erma is holding a cup of tea in a plastic, flesh coloured, spouted container given by staff. The lid is not on the right way. 11.45 she is still holding on to her cup, and the care staff have still not noticed that she cannot drink her tea. 11.50 Erma still has not drunk her tea, she is really trying hard to suck fluid out from the edge where the lid meets the cup. 11.55 no change. 12.00 no change. 12.05 she still tries to drink her tea but she cannot. She seems rather confused, she does not know what to do and needs someone to help her. At 12.25 Erma's cup of tea is now on the floor, a care assistant picks the cup up and takes it away. Erma did not drink any of the tea.

people at this home. They provide examples of some insights gained about individual people during mapping sessions, and the results were used to help the care provider gain a better understanding of the need for a different approach for different residents. The outcome of using Dementia Care Mapping in this context was to provide activities for no more than two or

Box 9.6

Notes from the DCM raw data sheet: 3/3/07 p.m.

A different mapper takes over in the afternoon and notes: Erma, lots of V [work-like activity], D [doing for self], Y [talking to an imaginary person] and T [sensory stimulation]. She has made several attempts to pick up the mug of tea that belongs to the lady next to her and finally manages this. She must be very thirsty – she drinks what is left in the cup and thoroughly enjoys it. This was recorded at 3.15 p.m., so Erma has waited all that time for a drink. Erma licks her glasses and smoothes her clothes. I feel worried that she cannot get out of her chair alone; she has made a few attempts and given up.

5.05 Erma is treated as an object, the chair moved to one side while she is still in it. Again, treated as an object during feeding; Erma can put her hand to her mouth and finger foods would be better than being spoon fed. During spoon feeding and again later, the pudding is served to the group at the table before Erma has finished her main course. Erma gets just left, several times during her meal, no explanation – while the careworker goes and does something else. Erma cannot recognise the cup with the spout, and anyway she is able to drink out of a mug (see notes at 3.15). This is a form of disempowerment. Finally a drink is poured down her even though she can lift a drink to her mouth if she is helped to start off the action.

three people at a time, and to take into account each person's individual capacity for doing.

In Box 9.4, evaluation of Janet's experience in the home tells us firstly that she has an inherent capacity for engaging with her world. However, in the absence of another person or tasks or objects to set the scene for pleasurable occupation, she slides into a state of disengagement. Following this evaluation, the staff now involve Janet in lunchtime preparation and take care to place objects within her environment such as a broom, books, flowers, so that she can happily 'potter' when the impulse to 'do' arises within her.

Boxes 9.5 and 9.6 give a little story of Erma's final triumph in getting some refreshment, and of her need for objects within her environment. The following day, as a result of feedback to staff about Erma's plight, a 'pat mat' was introduced to Erma. This is a clear plastic case, pillow shaped, filled with water and interesting shapes and colours. She tried to pick up the coloured stones and put them in her mouth; her instinct is to put things in her mouth. She touched the 'pat mat' and so I left it on the table next to her. It seemed to have a positive effect in that her repetitive behaviour gradually reduced; she was aware of its presence – she tentatively touched it and looked at it a few times. As time went on, her engagement with it increased and she became more confident. Within half an hour her behaviour had changed from a vacuous repetitive self-stimulation to a definite level of interest and a smiling disposition.

This close observation helped the staff group to understand how important objects are to her. In the absence of objects within her visual field and within reach, Erma loses her sense of self and engages in repetitive self-stimulation. Objects clearly help her to make the distinction between self and environment. She also needs help to start off actions such as drinking, even though she can grasp a mug. Without help, she is at risk of dehydrating. Furthermore, Erma received more negative interventions than any other resident. Using the DCM method helped staff to recognise and review these things and to take steps to tackle their own habitual practices.

Dementia Care Mapping has been found to be less helpful generally as a tool for monitoring the wellbeing and ill-being of those with severe dementia. Dementia Care Mapping deals primarily in behavioural composites, such as eating a meal, walking across a room, talking to another person – behaviours which are in fact an amalgam of many smaller components. It is therefore most effective in monitoring those people who are still able to live their lives in the context of such composites. It does not deal in behavioural *components* such as facial expression or gesture or eye contact, actions which are in fact retained long after the composite skill has disappeared.

The Positive Response Schedule (PRS)

The Positive Response Schedule (Perrin 1997a) is a system of direct observation which has been designed as a complement to Dementia Care Mapping for use with people who have severe dementia. It monitors (as far as is possible in severe dementia) levels of wellbeing, and may be used to measure the impact upon wellbeing of different therapeutic interventions, social interactions or environmental circumstances. The PRS operates in the context of single system methodology.

Single system methodology is not a standardised assessment or evaluation tool; that is, it does not generally measure a person's responses against a standardised set of criteria, as all the other instruments described in this chapter do. It may use one, as the Positive Response Schedule does, but it does not need one in order to function as a highly sensitive measure. Single system evaluation is a methodology which allows us to investigate the question, 'What specific interventions produce specific changes in specific individuals under specific conditions?'. It functions in the repeated collection of information on a single system over time, that system being an individual, a family, a group or other collective which is treated as a single unit (Bloom & Fischer 1982). Information is gathered through the sequential application and withdrawal or variation of an intervention, and the use of frequent, repeated outcome measures. Single system methodology is an immensely versatile means of assessing the impact of our interventions in dementia care. By way of example, it has been used to measure (Perrin 1996, 1997b):

- changes in wellbeing during massage, music, conversation, baking
- the effects of engagement in occupation on repetitive shouting
- improvements in spatial orientation following a personalised reorientation programme
- improvements in the recall of personal information
- independence in dressing
- the effects of different occupations upon engagement.

The uniqueness of the individuals with whom we are concerned in dementia care, determines that our interventions will engage with a broad and diverse range of criteria: a challenging behaviour or self-injury, continence or mobility, orientation or memory, depression or social isolation, dressing or feeding. The list is a long one, but single system methodology enables us to apply controlled measures to the problem under investigation, and thereby to determine the impact of our interventions. It is another tool for the tool-kit, and one that has much to offer the practitioner concerned to implement a truly person-centred approach.

CONCLUSION

The foundation for good dementia care lies, we believe, in a profiling process that informs care providers about the person's capacity for doing, along with reliable methods for evaluating the interventions we use. Without these, we subject the people in our care to 'hit and miss' interventions, and this is professionally irresponsible. People who have dementia deserve access to specialised services so that their occupational capacity can be understood in order to achieve optimal wellbeing. The work involved is specialised and time consuming, but the rewards are far reaching, as we hope this chapter illustrates.

References

Allen C K 1985 Occupational therapy for psychiatric diseases: measurement and management of cognitive disabilities. Little, Brown, Boston

Allen C K 1990 Allen cognitive test manual (with kit included). S & S Worldwide, Colchester, CT

Allen C K, Earhart C A, Blue T 1992 Occupational therapy treatment goals for the physically and cognitively disabled. The American Occupational Therapy Association Inc., Rockville, MD

Bloom M, Fischer J 1982 Evaluating practice: guidelines for the accountable professional. Prentice-Hall, Hillsdale, NJ

Bradford Dementia Group 2005 DCM 8 User's Manual. University of Bradford, Bradford

Brooker D 2007 Person centred care: making services better. Bradford Dementia Group Good Practice Guides. Jessica Kingsley, London

Commission for Social Care Inspection 2007 A new outcomes framework for performance assessment of adult social care 2006–2007. Commission for Social Care Inspection, London

Conroy C 1996 Dementia care: keeping intact and in touch. Avebury, Aldershot, Hampshire

May H (2008) Person centred care planning. Bradford Dementia Group Good Practice Guides. Jessica Kingsley, London

Perrin T 1996 Problem behaviour and the care of elderly people. Winslow Press, Oxon

Perrin T 1997a The positive response schedule for severe dementia. Ageing & Mental Health 1(2):184–191

Perrin T 1997b The role and value of occupation in severe dementia. Unpublished PhD thesis, University of Bradford

Pool J 2007 The Pool Activity Level (PAL) Instrument for Occupational Profiling: A Practical Resource for Carers of People with Cognitive Impairment, 2nd edn. Jessica Kingsley, London

Twiss S 1997 The problem of moral responsibility in medicine. The Journal of Medicine and Philosophy 2(4):341

Chapter 10

The dementia therapist: a good enough mother?

It is perhaps something of an anomaly in today's world of remedial health care professions, that we do not hear the term dementia therapist. We have physiotherapists and occupational therapists and speech therapists and hearing therapists and psychotherapists and movement therapists. It sometimes seems as though there is a therapist for every impairment known to man. But we don't have dementia therapists. Why should this be?

We have wondered if the reason for this is actually a hangover from 'old culture' attitudes, and old-world emphases on the word and the concept of 'care'. Nowhere is the term 'care' more overworked than in the field of older people and people with dementia. The terms dementia care and dementia carer are common currency, as are elderly care, home care, respite care, day care, carers' support, etc., etc. And there is of course nothing inherently wrong in the use of these terms. It is not until we understand the term in contrast to the term 'therapy' that a question mark appears. For we don't have elderly therapy or home therapy or day therapy; neither do we have occupational care or speech care or psycho-care. Why not? Well, it all seems to hinge on a concept of potential for change. Generally speaking carers care, with no anticipation of response or change on the part of the one cared for. Care is, effectively, one-sided – a 'doing-to'. Therapists care, on the other hand, with every expectation of change in the one cared for. Therapy is reciprocal – a 'working-with'. Care ministers, and expects nothing of the cared-for. Therapy demands, and expects much of the cared-for. Therapy does not accept the status quo. Therapists work with a person towards change, improvement, growth, adaptation – and herein lies the difference.

Traditionally, the common view of infirmity in old age, and of dementia particularly, has been nihilistic and hopeless. It's the end of the road, the inexorable descent, the inevitable deterioration and demise. This was the old culture of understanding around late life and disorders of late life. Change, growth and adaptation were not expected; all that was required as infirmity took over was a 'doing-to', until the end. This of course is no longer a universally held view; the new culture of understanding has served to issue a major challenge to such a stagnant negativism, and it would probably be true to say that the prevailing view today is hopeful rather than hopeless, positive rather than negative, constructive rather than static.

Building then on this comparatively recent cultural shift, we would want to add a further challenge: that we actively embrace the terms 'dementia therapy' and 'dementia therapist', and if not the terms, at least the concepts. For there is a movement, a reciprocity, a dynamic about *therapy* that is lacking in *care*, and as the culture continues to evolve, it is movement and change which are going to take us forward.

What would be the role of a dementia therapist, and who would take such a title? Well, it is conceivable that anyone who has a sustained and direct involvement with a person with dementia could take such a title. We ourselves could probably legitimately take the title, for all of our work revolves around people with dementia. But then we would perhaps lose something of our specialism (or there would be a perceived loss from outside the field), for we are first and foremost occupational therapists; occupation is our contribution and complements that of other disciplines. The RMN or the social worker who manages a residential establishment would probably also want to retain their own distinctive title and specialism.

We have wondered if maybe this is a role and a title for those whom we currently most commonly call care assistants. Now we know of course that of the many thousands of people who hold that title across the country, a good proportion do just that – assist with care. But we know, too, that there is also a good proportion who do considerably more than just assist with care. We all know those who genuinely love and give of themselves in the service of those for whom they have responsibility – people who make mistakes to be sure (don't we all?), but people who thirst for knowledge, who avail themselves of every possible opportunity for training, and who turn a job into a vocation. And most of us in the professions feel distinctly embarrassed that this army of skilled and devoted people should not attract a title, status and salary commensurate with their abilities and the quality of their service. We believe that this undervalued and underpaid group are worthy of recognition, and have wondered if a new role of dementia therapist might redress the balance.

What shape would such a role take, and what skills would it require? In order to explore this a little further, we return to the work of Donald Winnicott – this time to his concept of the 'good-enough mother' (1968). This is a model for childhood wellbeing certainly, but one that has a distinct application to dementia care also.

We have discussed in Chapter 4 the notion of mothering as an important concept for dementia, particularly late stage dementia, and we want to expand upon that a little. We need first perhaps to reiterate that we use the terms 'mothering' and 'good-enough mother' to imply a style of approach rather than gender. As far as we are concerned, gender is not at issue here, though one might argue as to why we are therefore using a gender-laden term. The simple answer is because we find it helpful and challenging, and the one that best illuminates the potential of the dementia therapist role. There are those (Schaffer 1977) who believe that mother may be a person of either sex, that attachment, bonding and satisfactory child-rearing may be accomplished by any unrelated adult taking over a parental role, and is a matter of personality, not of biology. To some degree we go along with that; certainly empirical evidence seems to bear this out (Anderson et al 1981, Phillips et al 1987). Nevertheless we also incline to the Winnicottian view of mixed male and female elements in either sex, and different qualities to the male and female elements: pure female elements relating to 'being' and pure male elements relating to 'doing' – a view later supported by Lamb (1981). Our position (before we go on to define mothering a little more carefully) is that both men and women are capable of mothering, but that because of a weighting of female elements in women, those who are most likely to mother, and to mother well, will be women. The far greater proportion of female staff to male in most care settings would appear to support this idea.

So what do we mean by good-enough mothering? Phillips' commentary on Winnicott (1988) puts it into a nutshell for us. The task of the good-enough mother is to present the world to the infant in manageable doses. And the task of those who are in a position of helping mothers and infants is to protect this process. Let us look at those two statements separately, and in the light of dementia.

A good-enough mother presents the world to the infant in manageable doses. Winnicott's perception of the neonatal infant is that he is unable to perceive himself in any way distinct from his mother; he is merged with, one and the same. He is in a state of absolute dependence, with no means of control, and no way of knowing the quality of care he is receiving except insofar as he gains profit or suffers disturbance from it. He is, in this phase, in a condition of unintegration, or unconnected feeling states. Mother's task here is a holding task: that is, a repetitive handling, keeping warm, bathing, rocking, nursing, naming, which has the effect over time of gathering together all those disparate feelings and impressions into a unified whole. Only in holding is there safety and security.

> 'It is especially at the start that mothers are vitally important, and indeed it is a mother's job to protect her infant from complications that cannot yet be understood by the infant, and to go on steadily providing the simplified bit of the world which the infant, through her, comes to know ... Only on a basis of monotony can a mother profitably add richness.' (Winnicott 1945)

If the holding has been adequate and consistent, in due course the child begins to separate the 'not-me' from the 'me', and gradually to relinquish mother en route towards independence. But he still needs mother to have charge over the presentation of the small doses:

> 'sharing a specialized bit of the world ... keeping that bit small enough so that the child is not muddled, yet enlarging it so that the growing capacity of the child to enjoy the world is catered for'.

A good-enough mother is not a perfect mother – just an ordinary person doing ordinary things. Provided that she herself has had good mothering, and is not an emotionally damaged person, what she has and how she behaves towards her child, is deeply instinctual, and not to be learned from books. That's it really – in simplified terms.

> '... the whole procedure of infant care has as its main characteristic a steady presentation of the world to the infant. This is something that cannot be done by thought, nor can it be managed mechanically. It can only be done by continuous management by a human being who is consistently herself. There is no question of perfection here. Perfection belongs to machines: what the infant needs is just what he usually gets, the care and attention of someone who is going on being herself. This of course applies to fathers too.' (Winnicott 1963)

We believe that this, too, should be the whole procedure of dementia care: a steady presentation of the world to the person who has dementia; small manageable doses – small enough not to muddle, large enough to satisfy and be enjoyed; protection from complication; holding, handling, sharing. This is the fundamental role of the good-enough mother, or perhaps we should say the good-enough dementia therapist, who is not perfect, not special, just an ordinary person, doing what, on the whole, comes naturally and intuitively.

And what about our second proposition regarding good-enough mothering – that the task of those who help mothers and their children is to protect the process of presenting the world in manageable doses?

> 'If it be true, or even possible that the mental health of every individual is founded by the mother in her living experience with her infant, doctors and nurses can make it their first duty not to interfere. Instead of trying to teach mothers how to do what in fact cannot be taught, paediatricians must come sooner or later to recognize a good mother when they see one and then make sure that she gets full opportunity to grow into her job.' (Winnicott 1948)

What about those of us who oversee the appointment and the work of those we could call dementia therapists? Maybe this is our task too: to recognise those in whom the ability to hold and to handle in appropriate ways comes naturally, and when they are recognised, to ensure that they get full opportunity to grow into their job. Love and empathy cannot be taught. If they are not there, there is no book nor teaching method that will instil them; these are the basic prerequisites for any would-be dementia therapist. But if they *are* there, we can provide the growing medium which will shape and mould to the flowering of full potential.

That 'growing medium' will of course embrace guidance and tuition in some measure, but we are not asking our good-enough dementia therapist to go away and train for three years, nor to pass exams in health and social care, nor even necessarily to become vastly knowledgeable about dementia. We *are* asking that he or she will be a person committed to growing; in other words, we are asking that in addition to an inherent love and empathy, there will be an openness and ability to think and to reflect upon actions and experiences, and a willingness and ability to adapt accordingly. Strictly speaking, it is not possible to 'teach' any given individual how to present the world in manageable doses to any other; this is a knowledge and a skill which is in part instinctive and intuitive, and in part environmentally shaped. It is not possible to set standard guidelines for mothering; for every infant and every mother is unique, and therefore every relationship and interaction between the two will be unique. Nevertheless for those of us who are trainers and/or supervisors, an integral part of our commitment to those for whom we have responsibility, is to provide a model of good practice, to give permission to use the model, and to ensure that the model is understood.

So for example, most mothers know intuitively that a four-month-old should not be expected to use a knife and fork. Similarly, most people who work with late dementia also know intuitively that the person who has returned to an early developmental level should not be expected to use a knife and fork. But their instinctive response (to encourage that person to eat with their fingers) is often overridden by deeply inculcated 'old culture' messages about age-appropriateness, and the dignity of cleanliness and orderliness (see 'Helen' in Chapter 9). And so despite all that their 'gut response' tells them, they impart these ingrained attitudes and insist on the use of knife and fork, regardless of the impact upon the person with dementia. Our responsibility as trainers is to set our staff free from such constraints, and in order for this to take place some kind of formal training is without doubt necessary. It may be in the classroom, it may be in the workplace, it may be delivered as a lecture, it may be an informal giving of permission ('It's quite alright for Joan to use her fingers. Look, she is far less stressed when we let her do her own thing'). *How* this knowledge is imparted is immaterial; *that* it is imparted is crucial. For these are the parameters within which staff can work in comfort and in confidence, and which permit full expression of intuition and individuality. The setting of those parameters is our responsibility.

We would like to see the creation of a new role or new post of dementia therapist in residential and day care settings. This would not be for the person for whom this work is just a money-earner, nor for those who are simply content to 'do to' according to standardised policies and procedures. People such as these may justifiably retain the title of care assistant. But for those individuals who understand therapy as opposed to care, who have a commitment to 'working with', to 'making better', to a dynamic style of interaction and intervention which seeks change and growth, we believe that such a role would represent a re-evaluation and a revaluation of skills and expertise. We would see the creation of such a role as instigating a significant and much needed cultural shift in the dementia world. We recognise of course that this does rather go against the grain. Health care society has come to expect that anyone calling themselves a therapist will have done several years training and have at least a diploma, if not a degree. But we all know that degrees are no assurance of interpersonal skills. We have all come across the occasional therapist of one discipline or another who has a higher degree and not the first idea of how to engage with people. And yet this person commands a status and a salary that a care assistant at Dunroamin Nursing Home can only dream about. There is something very wrong here. We believe that a new role of dementia therapist for appropriately qualified people (qualified by personal calibre not by degree), attracting responsibility and enhanced financial reward, will make a significant difference to the quality of dementia services currently offered.

The situation that we have currently in our care homes and day centres across the country, is a barely perceptible but nevertheless inexorable leaching out of high calibre people into other jobs, professional training or management positions – not because they do not care for the work, but because they cannot command a living wage, achieve due status or acquire responsibility in any other way. The sad reality is that very many of those currently holding the position of care assistant have come to the work from school, from 'non-people' jobs, or from raising a family, patiently serve a long apprenticeship in which they develop an extensive range of skills and expertise, become dissatisfied and devalued by a wage and a status that bears no resemblance to their qualities and their commitment, and leave – usually at the peak of their influence and efficiency. And the dementia world continues to muddle along in a state of perpetual impoverishment. Only as we learn to value and reward the expertise of our personnel in tangible and substantial ways, as some other sectors of society do, are we going to see improvement in our dementia services of any real substance and significance.

So it may be that what we have proposed resonates with others in the field and a new role comes into being. But whether it does or it doesn't, there is a sense in which all of us who work with people with dementia are dementia therapists (or should be). For the task for us all, no matter of what discipline, is that indicated above – presenting the world to our client in manageable doses. That's what it's all about really, when it's boiled down to its lowest common denominator. It sounds so simple, but of course it isn't. It is highly skilled, very specialised work in which therapeutic success or failure hinge entirely upon the qualities and abilities of the therapist. So as we start to draw this text to a close, it is probably worth recapping and reaffirming those therapeutic attributes which are needed to carry out such a task.

A good-enough dementia therapist needs:

- to retain an openness about the nature and causes of dementia itself, and to recognise a distinct psychosocial element to its cause, course and manifestation
- to understand the occupational nature of people, and occupation itself as a prime target of therapeutic intervention
- to appreciate the importance of wellbeing over function as the focus for intervention
- to recognise the decline of dementia as broadly analogous to childhood developmental processes in reverse, and thereby to understand that the person in later dementia inhabits a world which is very different to that which we inhabit
- to understand the critical importance of the therapeutic relationship to therapeutic efficacy, and to the wellbeing of the person with dementia
- to appreciate the significance of playfulness in the therapeutic relationship, and to develop a playful approach
- to bring an individualised, multifaceted, non-prescriptive approach to assessment and intervention

- to recognise the changes in thinking and doing that take place within a person's experience over the course of their dementia, and to be able to adapt occupational interventions accordingly
- to make a commitment to learning the language of dementia
- to develop such a knowledge of each individual's world, and the changing picture of that world over time, that the apportioning of 'manageable bits' of the world as we know it, is executed judiciously and proficiently.

This is good enough. More than good enough in fact. The person who is able to fulfil these criteria, or at least to grow towards these criteria, is the person who will take forward the quality of service provision for people with dementia into a new era. Those of us in the field in positions of management, staff supervision and education have two prime tasks. First, we need to seek and employ people having those fundamental 'building block' qualities of love, compassion and empathy, and, where possible, to let go those who haven't. The second task is then to provide that growing medium which will enable them to realise their full potential. Conventional training methods are but one constituent of that growing medium. The greater and most effective part is actually a 'showing by doing' – an apprenticeship model. Mothers mother, by and large, in the way that they themselves were mothered; they learned by example, good or bad. It is not so very different for carers and therapists. If our staff are not yet good enough therapists, if they are not yet fulfilling the criteria set out above, then maybe it is a salutary exercise to look at our own practice. Are we good enough? Are we proficient in therapeutic endeavour? Those we teach, whether by didactic method or by hands-on demonstration, will reflect what we are.

This is perhaps a salutary consideration, for those we now teach may well be mothering us in the not too distant future; we may be finding ourselves at the sharp end of their care or therapeutic intervention. We are of an age where we cannot deny the imminence or the reality of our own ageing, or the potential of a dementing process within our own personal experience. It might not happen; but it might, and it would be folly not to give the possibility some consideration. Who will care for us, and what will be the quality of what they have to offer? The future is ours – it is an awesome responsibility.

References

Anderson C, Nagle R, Roberts W, Smith J 1981 Attachment to substitute caregivers as a function of center quality and caregiver involvement. Child Development 52:53–61

Lamb M 1981 The development of father–infant relationships. In: Lamb M (ed) The role of the father in child development. Wiley, New York

Phillips A 1988 Winnicott. Fontana, London

Phillips D, McCartney K, Scarr S 1987 Child care quality and children's social development. Developmental Psychology 23:537–543

Schaffer R 1977 Mothering. Fontana, Glasgow

Winnicott D 1945 Primitive emotional development. In: Winnicott D 1958 Collected papers: through paediatrics to psycho-analysis. Tavistock, London

Winnicott D 1948 Paediatrics and psychiatry. In: Winnicott D 1958 Collected papers: through paediatrics to psycho-analysis. Tavistock, London

Winnicott D 1963 From dependence towards independence in the development of the individual. In: Winnicott D 1965 The maturational processes and the facilitating environment: studies in the theory of emotional development. Hogarth Press, London

Winnicott D 1968 Communication between infant and mother, and mother and infant, compared and contrasted. In: Winnicott D 1987 Babies and their mothers. Free Association Books, London

Index